Establishing a Healthcare Emergency Response Coalition

JAY LEE,
THOMAS W. CLEARE,
AND MARY RUSSELL

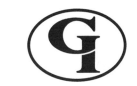

GOVERNMENT INSTITUTES
An imprint of
THE SCARECROW PRESS, INC.
Lanham • Toronto • Plymouth, UK
2010

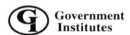
Government Institutes

Published by Government Institutes
An imprint of The Scarecrow Press, Inc.
A wholly owned subsidary of The Rowman & Littlefield Publishing Group, Inc.
4501 Forbes Boulevard, Suite 200, Lanham, Maryland 20706
http://www.govinstpress.com

Estover Road, Plymouth PL6 7PY, United Kingdom

British Library Cataloguing in Publication Information Available

Library of Congress Cataloging-in-Publication Data

Lee, Jay, 1948–2010
  Establishing a healthcare emergency response coalition / Jay Lee, Thomas W. Cleare, and Mary Russell.
    p. ; cm.
  Includes bibliographical references and index.
  ISBN 978-1-60590-680-5 (pbk. : alk. paper)
 1. Emergency medical services—United States—Planning. 2. Disaster medicine—United States—Planning.
3. Coalitions. I. Cleare, Thomas W., 1970– II. Russell, Mary, 1953– III. Government Institutes. IV. Title.
  [DNLM: 1. Emergency Medical Services. 2. Community Health Planning. 3. Disaster Planning. 4. Health Care Coalitions—organization & administration. WX 215 L478e 2010]
  RA645.5.L44 2010
  362.18—dc22

2010014763

Printed in the United States of America

Dedicated to
Benjamin ("Jay") Youngblood Lee

As director for disaster services at the Palm Beach County Medical Society, Jay Lee contributed to the development of this book, but sadly passed away on February 4, 2010. His professionalism, dedication, and sense of humor will be dearly missed by all who worked with him at the local, regional, state, and national level.

Contents

Acknowledgments

Special thanks go to the board of directors and the leadership team at the Palm Health-care Foundation, Inc., for their financial support in making the Healthcare Emergency Response Coalition of Palm Beach County, Florida, a reality. In addition, the formation of the Healthcare Emergency Response Coalition (HERC) would not have been possible without the vision and persistence of Dr. Jeff Davis, the former medical director for the Health Care District of Palm Beach County, and the Palm Beach County Medical Services Society board of directors and Executive Director Tenna Wiles. Special appreciation also to Craig DeAtley at the Institute for Public Health Emergency Readiness, Washington Hospital Center, for his consulting and guidance in the development of HERC.

HERC has been extremely fortunate in its leaders. We particularly wish to acknowledge and thank the HERC chairpersons who have served through the years: William Farrell, Alfred Grasso, Mary Russell, Robbin Lee, Cindy Lang, and Michael Self. We would also like to acknowledge the many individuals who have donated their time and knowledge by serving on the executive steering committee and the other HERC standing committees.

Finally, we are extremely appreciative of our twenty-two core member organizations for their continued commitment to HERC in meeting its mission to develop and promote the healthcare emergency preparedness and response and recovery capability of Palm Beach County, Florida:

A. G. Holley Hospital
American Red Cross
Bethesda Memorial Hospital
Boca Raton Community Hospital
Columbia Hospital
Delray Medical Center
Good Samaritan Medical Center
Health Care District of Palm Beach
  County
JFK Medical Center
Jupiter Medical Center
Lakeside Medical Center

Palm Beach County Department of
  Emergency Management
Palm Beach County Fire Rescue
Palm Beach County Health Department
Palm Beach County Medical Society Services
Palm Beach County Sheriff's Office
Palm Beach Gardens Medical Center
Palms West Hospital
St. Mary's Medical Center
VA Medical Center
Wellington Regional Medical Center
West Boca Medical Center

Introduction

From big cities to small rural towns, all communities can be vulnerable to emergencies, disasters, and even catastrophes. There have been a number of events in the United States and abroad demonstrating the surge on the healthcare system from those who are injured or ill. Terrorist attacks, bombings, weather events, wildfires, structural collapse, and most recently the H1N1 pandemic all have impacted hospitals and other healthcare system facilities.

Big cities are not the only communities vulnerable to mass casualty events. In 2001, while big cities like New York City and Washington, D.C., experienced catastrophic healthcare events, the small rural community of Stonycreek Township in Pennsylvania found itself vulnerable as well. While there were no survivors on United Airlines Flight 93, the location of the crash provided a clear reminder that mass casualty events do not discriminate based on the size of the community. Also in 2001, the midsize city of Boca Raton, Florida, found itself in the middle of a serious healthcare event. This is where the first of several anthrax-tainted letters was received, which resulted in the first anthrax-related fatality associated with the 2001 letters.

Natural disasters can also cause major surges on the healthcare system. From earthquakes across California to tornadoes stretching from South Dakota through Nebraska, Kansas, Oklahoma, Texas, and the surrounding areas known as Tornado Alley, Mother Nature can strike without warning and leave thousands injured and even knock hospitals out of service for extended periods. Even with prior warning, hurricanes can inflict severe damage across both small rural communities and big cities. Florida has long experienced healthcare needs associated with hurricanes, with the best-known striking the southeast Florida coast in 1992 known as Hurricane Andrew. In 2005 Hurricane Katrina made landfall at the small town of Buras-Triumph, Louisiana, ravaging the coasts of Louisiana, Alabama, and Mississippi and inflicting severe damage throughout the three states and surrounding areas. In New Orleans, hospitals and nursing homes were isolated and cut off from rescuers for extended periods of time. The catastrophic healthcare event surrounding Katrina once again demonstrated that all communities, regardless of size and location, can be vulnerable to mass casualty events that will stress and even break the best healthcare system.

Natural and man-made disasters are not the only types of events that can challenge the healthcare system of a community. Pandemics, disease outbreaks, and seasonal health issues can also stress a hospital's or healthcare organization's ability to respond to the needs of a community. The H1N1 flu, the "bird" flu, West Nile virus, seasonal flu, and norovirus, as well as many other disease outbreaks, can all provide a surge of patients to a hospital that can stress its capacity and capabilities.

How should a community and its healthcare system prepare for a major healthcare event? This book presents the coalition model as a framework for bringing together the healthcare community, fire rescue, law enforcement, and emergency management to address the preparedness needs of a community. The recommendation to utilize the coalition organizational structure is supported nationally. Findings from a study commissioned by the U.S. Department of Health and Human Services (HHS) found that healthcare coalitions have emerged throughout the United States.[1] Based on the findings from the HHS study, a 2009 recommendation proposed that "healthcare coalitions should become the foundation of a national strategy for healthcare preparedness and response for catastrophic health events."[2]

OVERVIEW OF THE BOOK

This book is designed as a working guidebook to allow community stakeholders to walk through the process of establishing a healthcare emergency response coalition for their community. Work assignments are provided throughout each chapter that will prompt readers to answer questions, make lists, and brainstorm ideas for their community.

Chapter 1 begins with an overview of the coalition organizational structure and how the coalition model can prove to be a good framework for multiple organizations to work collectively on challenges facing a community. Chapter 1 will start readers thinking about the types of challenges they need to prepare for and the types of stakeholders that should be brought together to plan for and address the challenges.

Chapter 2 dives right in to the importance of a healthcare emergency response coalition. Readers will review how healthcare coalitions can help with Joint Commission, regulatory compliance, hazard vulnerability assessments, community-wide exercises and drills, training, and other valuable resources coalitions can bring to members.

Chapter 3 reviews some different approaches to healthcare emergency response coalitions by examining how coalitions in several communities are structured. The HERC of Palm Beach County, Florida, is examined in greater detail, identifying the factors that led to its creation and how the coalition brings value to its members.

Chapter 4 presents readers with ideas on how to structure a healthcare emergency response coalition. Examples of how to bring key stakeholders together, how to enlist support from CEOs, and how to choose a fiscal agent for the coalition are reviewed in detail. Desired qualities of the coalition leader are presented, and the many administrative tasks necessary to operate a coalition are reviewed.

Chapter 5 walks readers through the important steps of establishing goals, implementing objectives, and establishing emergency response procedures. This process is presented as a strategic planning exercise, in which strengths, weaknesses, opportunities, and threats are identified and coalition members develop the key objectives and action items for the coalition. The very important standardized emergency response procedures are presented, with the encouragement that the coalition collectively develop, approve, and implement a standardized set of training protocols.

Chapter 6 reviews ways to sustain a coalition once it has been established. Funding alternatives are identified, along with activities that can be undertaken to garner and maintain support from leaders of the respective coalition members.

Chapter 7 provides a summary in the format of a top-ten list identifying tips that are important for successful coalition building. This chapter provides readers with an opportunity to revisit some of the critical components presented throughout the book.

The appendixes provide information taken directly from an established HERC including a sample Memorandum of Agreement, Operational Guidelines and a Strategic Plan. Additional copies of administrative forms, joint exercise plans, and reports can be obtained by request at:

Attention: Healthcare Emergency Response Coalition
c/o Palm Beach County Medical Society Services
3540 Forest Hill Boulevard, Suite 101
West Palm Beach, Florida 33406
Phone: 561-433-3940
www.pbcms.org/herc

NOTES

1. E. Toner, R. Waldhorn, C. Franco, B. Courtney, A. Norwood, K. Rambhia, T. V. Inglesby, and T. O'Toole, *Hospitals Rising to the Challenge: The First Five Years of the U.S. Hospital Preparedness Program and Priorities Going Forward,* prepared by the Center for Biosecurity of UPMC for the U.S. Department of Health and Human Services under Contract No. HHSO100200700038C. 2009.

2. B. Courtney, E. Toner, R. Waldhorn, C. Franco, K. Rambhia, A. Norwood, T. V. Inglesby, and T. O'Toole, "Healthcare Coalitions: The New Foundation for National Healthcare Preparedness and Response for Catastrophic Health Emergencies," *Biosecurity and Bioterrorism: Biodefense Strategy, Practice, and Science* 7, no. 2 (July 2009): 117–123.

1

Why Start a Healthcare Emergency Response Coalition?

Healthcare organizations, whether they are hospitals, physician practices, nursing homes, or one of the many other types of healthcare entities, are often faced with challenges that are too big to be addressed alone. These large, often community-wide challenges require the concerted effort of the healthcare community. In this book, the types of challenges discussed center on natural and man-made disasters, terrorist attacks, pandemics, and mass casualty events. To address these challenges, the flexible organizational structure known as coalitions is presented as a proven model to address community-wide challenges by bringing together the healthcare community to work in partnership with the many emergency response agencies found in a community. This multidisciplinary approach includes the many healthcare disciplines along with law enforcement, fire rescue, public health, and emergency management, among others.

UNDERSTANDING COALITIONS

When faced with a community-wide challenge, individual organizations often find that a collective approach to meeting such a challenge is more advantageous than proceeding independently. By definition, a community-wide challenge impacts all organizations within a geographic area, sparing none. The unique nature of such a challenge suspends the constraints of competition and frees organizations to work together on a unified approach to foster benefits for all organizations. The ability to leverage resources by combining the expertise of multiorganization staff and the ability to share the financial burden of such an endeavor can provide individual organizations with a return on their "investment" that far outweighs their contribution.

How do organizations come together to tackle a community-wide challenge? They do so collaboratively, by partnering with one another and forming a coalition. Coalitions can be a very flexible organizational structure for ongoing projects, involving members from separate organizations. Coalitions do not require formal filings or other instruments of legal establishment. Functioning as an interacting group of individuals from multiple organizations, coalitions are deliberately constructed, lack internal structure, have mutually perceived membership, and are focused on goals requiring concerted member action.[1]

ACTION-ORIENTED GROUPS

Coalitions are often some of the most effective and productive groups. Since collaborative goals and objectives guide the work of the coalition members, almost all efforts are directed at the desired outcome. The concentrated focus inherent in coalition activities enables coalitions to be action-oriented groups. Simply stated, coalitions exist to get a job done.

Ideally, coalitions comprise individuals who have the autonomy to work on a project without close direction. As a result, the individual members of a coalition can collectively agree upon the work to be done and then carry out whatever tasks are necessary without the need for supervisory approval. This unique characteristic of coalitions distinguishes them from the more bureaucratic structure found in many formal organizations.

EVOLUTION OF A COALITION

Coalitions typically start from small groups of individuals who come together to address an issue that none of the individuals are in a position to address by themselves. This could range from a coalition internal to an organization to a coalition comprising members from separate organizations. The common element is that the members of a coalition all face a common challenge and collectively agree that they would like to work together in partnership to accomplish their objectives.

As coalitions accomplish some of their initial goals, the members quickly recognize the effectiveness of the structure. This performance or outcome-related affirmation helps drive coalition members to improve on their initial work or expand into related projects that bring additional value to their organizations and the community. Occasionally, the success of a coalition can lead to the formation of a nonprofit organization to carry on the original work of the group in a more formalized capacity.

HOW HEALTHCARE COALITIONS CAN ACCOMPLISH COLLABORATIVE OBJECTIVES

Hospitals, physicians, and other healthcare providers are trained, staffed, and equipped to independently handle both routine and complicated medical cases, tend to accident victims, and address just about any clinical challenge that presents. However, there are situations in which even the best and best-equipped healthcare organizations will find it difficult to deliver care. For example, the volume of cases from a mass casualty event may easily stress the emergency-department capacity of a hospital and its physicians. A natural disaster like a hurricane can knock out power, shut down transportation routes, and leave a hospital functioning in isolation for an undetermined period of time. A terrorist attack on an underground subway system could expose hundreds of passengers to a biological substance and quickly overwhelm even the largest healthcare system with patients in need of decontamination, evaluation, and treatment. Each of these crises and many more similar events require a collaborative and multidisciplinary approach to manage.

The healthcare coalition structure is an organizational model that can be used to address both big and small problems facing a community. The coalition structure allows hospitals, physicians, nursing homes, dialysis providers, home health agencies, and other providers to work together across organizational lines to prepare for and address critical challenges facing a community. If hospitals and nursing homes plan and work together, they can more effectively address the many unforeseen dilemmas that can arise as a hurricane approaches a community. Pharmacies and physicians who plan together can ensure that patients have the appropriate amount of medication to last through a disaster event. Hospitals and physicians that train together can help ensure that patients in any kind of mass casualty event receive the appropriate decontamination, evaluation, and treatment. Through this interorganizational collaboration, healthcare coalitions can accomplish many collaborative objectives.

Considering the challenges your organization faces, list at least three examples of issues that a coalition of stakeholders could work together to address.

_____

_____

_____

_____

_____

_____

_____

_____

_____

_____

_____

_____

_____

HEALTHCARE COALITIONS MAXIMIZE INCLUSION IN SYSTEM PLANNING, RESPONSE, AND RECOVERY

The healthcare coalition structure demonstrates a willingness by the healthcare community to come to the table as a partner to address the many challenges a community might face. As a result, coalitions enable the healthcare community to partner with the emergency preparedness community to optimally prepare for all challenges. For example, a coalition can bring together all the hospitals in a region, the physician community, representatives from nursing homes, and other healthcare providers to work hand in hand with fire rescue, law enforcement, the local public health agency, and emergency management.

When the collaborative objective is related to emergency preparedness, evidence demonstrates that all stakeholders who will be involved in the response to a disaster event should plan and train together. By working together in a coalition structure, representatives from multiple organizations and multiple disciplines can implement unified training protocols, common communication systems, and most importantly, build relationships with the colleagues who will be responding to an event. The coalition that includes the emergency response partners will help ensure that the healthcare community is included in the overall system planning, response, and recovery operations.

What types of disciplines or professions should be represented in your healthcare coalition?

_____

_____

_____

_____

_____

_____

_____

_____

_____

_____

_____

_____

_____

_____

_____

COMMUNITY SUPPORT

When a group of hospitals, physicians, and other healthcare providers come together to form a coalition, it enables them to generate additional support from the community. Local governments and emergency response professionals are often motivated to leverage their resources to help further expand hospital, physician, and provider capabilities to respond to a disaster event. Local and state politicians are better positioned to bring resources to a community when they can demonstrate a true collaborative approach through a coalition. In addition, local and national foundations often find that large groups partnering together can maximize their grant dollars, as opposed to single entities working on more narrow projects. The coalition structure can be used to foster greater community support to address the challenges that healthcare organizations face on a daily basis.

List community leaders outside of the coalition who could be called upon to enlist community support for your coalition's efforts.

_____

_____

_____

_____

_____

_____

_____

_____

_____

_____

_____

_____

_____

NOTE

1. W. B. Stevenson, J. L. Pearce, et al., "The Concept of 'Coalition' in Organization Theory and Research," *Academy of Management Review* 10, no. 2 (1985): 256–268.

2

The Importance of Healthcare Emergency Response Coalitions

Hospitals are recognized as critical infrastructure within their communities as they provide around-the-clock services during times of everyday emergencies and disasters. There is an inherent responsibility to comply with emergency management standards and recommendations from a number of agencies and to be prepared to manage all kinds of incidents that may range from simple to catastrophic. This all-hazards scalable approach involves training in the national incident management system (NIMS) and the national response framework and using a hospital incident command system approach.

NATIONAL AGENCIES THAT PROVIDE EMERGENCY MANAGEMENT GUIDANCE FOR HOSPITALS:

- Centers for Disease Control and Prevention (CDC), www.cdc.gov
- Department of Health and Human Services (HHS), www.hhs.gov
- Department of Homeland Security (DHS), www.dhs.gov
- Environmental Protection Agency (EPA), www.epa.gov
- Federal Emergency Management Agency (FEMA), www.fema.gov
- The Joint Commission, www.jointcommission.org
- National Fire Protection Association (NFPA), www.nfpa.org
- National Institute for Occupational Safety and Health (NIOSH), www.cdc.gov/niosh
- Occupational Safety and Health Administration (OSHA), www.osha.gov

---

Communities also have state standards to follow, such as from the department of health, in addition to local planning guidelines, such as from the local emergency planning committee, their local emergency operations center, the county public health department, and others.

Hospitals are encouraged to collaborate with community partners and to conduct joint planning, utilize interoperable communications, integrate their command structure during a response, develop contingencies when utilities or supply issues occur, and participate in exercises and after-action reviews that include local emergency management and response agencies.

Prior to the formation of the HERC in Palm Beach County, the healthcare community was similar to most other communities: highly challenged to address emergency preparedness in a collaborative and integrated manner.

Local disasters have a way of serving as a wake-up call. In Florida, this occurred when Hurricane Andrew made landfall in 1992 on the lower Florida southeast coast as a Category 5 storm. There had not been a major storm in a twenty-five-year prior period of time. The storm caused significant community infrastructure damage and disruption, including loss of power and water and building damage to healthcare facilities, businesses, and employee homes. Patients were evacuated to other hospitals and mutual aid was needed for months. The recovery process took years to complete.

The terrorist attacks on the World Trade Center in 1993 and the sequence of tragic events on September 11, 2001, generated a new level of awareness of intentional threats. The anthrax mailings in October 2001, including those within Palm Beach County, Florida, increased the concern of both the public and healthcare agencies about preparedness for such events.

An influx of federal funding to public health helped pay for equipment purchases, administrative support, and expanded training efforts. Hospitals received Health Resources and Services Administration (HRSA) money to help with their bioterrorism preparedness efforts. Agencies found the funding was helpful; however, the following issues were noted:

- Individual agencies worked independently and at times competitively.
- Training was accomplished by each hospital individually, and there was inconsistency in the curriculum between facilities.
- Planning and response terminology was inconsistent across agencies.
- Personnel linkages and networking among the healthcare community was extremely limited.
- Response procedures were developed without knowledge or input from respective agencies that could possibly be impacted.
- Communication interoperability between responders was minimal and there was a lack of information-sharing strategies.
- There was a minimum of integration of health and medical assets into the public safety response.
- Many important timely issues were not being addressed at all.
- The public had little knowledge of efforts to protect the community and resultant benefits to boost their confidence.

A disaster event serves as a definite motivator for healthcare agencies to consider working together more effectively, especially if the threat is one that has a potential for recurrence.

Natural disasters are a good example of recurrent threats; this could mean hurricanes in Florida, earthquakes and wildfires in California, tornadoes in the Midwest, and blizzards in the Northeast.

As part of an accreditation requirement and to meet state and federal emergency management standards, hospitals conduct an annual hazard vulnerability analysis (HVA) to rank a list of hazards, the probability of their occurrence, the impact they might have, and the preparedness level and capability of the hospital to manage such threats, internally and with external community partners. The HVA process is to be conducted with local emergency management and response partners. Both sudden-impact and developing-impact disaster scenarios need to be considered.

There is also a need to examine the capacity and capability of healthcare agencies to manage disasters that have various levels of magnitude and the scalability of an emergency response. Catastrophic planning is recommended to be conducted as a multiagency endeavor to integrate planning and response efforts among local, regional, state, and federal agencies.

The Department of Homeland Security has developed a list of fifteen national planning scenarios, fourteen of which apply to hospitals.[1] Most of these could result in the potential for a surge of casualties, some requiring specific capabilities for hospitals to be able to manage:

- Aerosol anthrax
- Blister agent
- Chlorine tank explosion
- Cyberattack
- Food contamination
- Improvised explosive device (IED)
- Improvised nuclear device (IND)
- Major earthquake
- Major hurricane
- Nerve agent
- Pandemic influenza
- Plague
- Radiological dispersal device (RDD)
- Toxic industrial chemicals

The national planning scenarios are to be considered in addition to other potential disaster threats that can cause mass casualties, including the following:

Weather:
- Hail/ice storm
- Severe cold
- Severe heat
- Severe rain/flooding
- Snowstorm
- Tornado

Security:
- Bomb
- Civil disturbance
- Gang violence
- Hostage situation
- School shooting

Utility failures:
- Electrical
- Emergency generator
- Fire suppression/alarms
- Fuel (diesel, propane, butane, natural gas)
- Heating/ventilation/air cooling
- Information systems
- Medical vacuum
- Overhead paging
- Oxygen
- Security and access control
- Sewer
- Telephone/telecommunications
- Water main break/low water pressure

Transportation:
- Airplane crash
- Highway (car/truck/bus)
- Rail crash

Structural:
- Bridge collapse
- Chemical/hazmat spill/release
- Damage to building
- Explosion
- Fire
- Gas leak

What hazards exist in your area that are recurrent and scalable (ranging from mild to catastrophic)?

_____

_____

_____

_____

_____

_____

_____

_____

_____

_____

_____

_____

_____

BENEFITS OF A HEALTHCARE EMERGENCY RESPONSE COALITION

Coalitions provide an efficient mechanism to accomplish common goals among health-care partners through the continuum of planning and preparedness before events occur, response during events, and recovery after events have occurred. Examples in which working together as a healthcare emergency response coalition for preparedness, response, and recovery include the following.

Communications

Coalitions can select and use common systems for threat notification, activations, and routine sharing of information about meetings, training, and resources. Generating a common contact list with facility 24/7 command center and HERC membership contact information including e-mail, phone, cell numbers and pagers, Blackberries, or beepers allows for rapid dissemination of critical information. Many hospitals are now using event management software systems that allow storage of contact and resource numbers; however, key contact information also needs to be shared with local emergency management in the event of a sudden-impact incident. Reporting of bed availability per county, region, or state requests can be completed electronically; however, hospitals need to be issued login and password information well ahead of any incidents. Common communications systems can be purchased with group pricing to minimize cost, with shared training sessions and exercises to ensure that facility representatives can use the equipment, participate in weekly roll-calls, and be operational in a disaster. Local emergency management has communication subject matter experts that can support hospitals with programming of critical channels for interoperability with emergency response partners. The local emergency operations center will activate its joint information center during a major disaster. This resource supports the release of credible, consistent emergency messaging across all agencies and reduces the burden of individual hospitals to develop their own press releases during a major disaster.

Training

Coalitions can support shared training sessions for core competencies such as disaster awareness, operations-level training, decontamination, use of communication systems, community mass care management, critical infrastructure assessment and protection, risk communications, disaster behavioral health training, continuity of operations planning (COOP), and a range of others that are all-hazards or hazard-specific. Examples of hazard-specific courses include incident command system classroom training, radiological awareness and operations-level training, hazardous waste operations and emergency response (HAZWOPER), biological disaster preparation, response and recovery, county points of distribution and staging areas, and laboratory packing and shipping standards, among others. Support for general training needs such as grant writing and grant management sessions are also very helpful when conducted with multiple hospitals at once. State partners issuing grants are grateful to have a consolidated session to attend, and participants feel supported in understanding expectations and understanding requirements for deliverables for all awardees.

Exercises

Hospitals can voluntarily choose to participate in a scheduled range of community-wide, regional, or statewide exercises that are Homeland Security Exercise and Evaluation Program (HSEEP) compliant. This can include seminars, workshops, tabletop exercises, drills, and functional or full-scale exercises. Emergency management typically will use their planners and experts to develop the master scenario events list (MSEL), enlist agencies to participate, and facilitate after-action reviews, which can be quite time-consuming and beyond the resource capabilities of individual hospitals. The coalition can generate a list of objectives that are hospital or healthcare group–specific, in addition to each hospital adding objectives that they specifically need to test. Typically, each coalition will identify an exercise committee that actively participates in the joint planning sessions with emergency management and response partners.

Joint Planning

Planning can be all-hazards or hazard-specific, and coalitions can benefit from comprehensive emergency management planning with their local emergency management and emergency response partners. Traditional partners include law enforcement, fire rescue, and public health. Nontraditional partners include supply vendors, partners within the continuum of care (hospice, long-term care, funeral homes), dialysis centers, blood banks, mental health centers, and others. By communicating information about capacity and capability, there is a shared understanding of how partners will need to respond to support each other.

An example might be a hospital that is located near a large university. Planning will include methods of communication for incidents, plan of action for security, access control, on-site treatment areas, next-of-kin notification, and other concerns. This will help alleviate fears by the hospital that it will suddenly be surged with hundreds of students, whether a school shooting has occurred or there is an outbreak of biological illness. Universities also need to communicate hazardous materials, location, and quantities maintained on campus for classroom or research work, and this is included as part of the HVA risk assessment to be communicated to the hospital, among other response partners. Joint planning with universities and encouraging them to participate in coalition meetings helps support the training needs of healthcare agencies. Some universities have simulation research centers that include disaster skills training for biomedical students, local healthcare professionals, and as primary or refresher training for medical reserve corps members.

Planning needs to include triggers to adapt a response according to the scale of a disaster. Florida considers hurricanes to be a priority hazard that tends to be recurrent and requires scalability of the response needed according to the anticipated category of storm per the Saffir-Simpson scale. The numerous storms that tracked through the state during 2004–2005 prompted multiagency catastrophic planning, including health and medical representatives from local hospitals and healthcare facilities, and state and federal agencies. Catastrophic planning within coalitions can include patient evacuation scenarios from multiple facilities. This of course is linked with patient tracking and transportation asset assignments. Working with local emergency management through the Emergency Support Function 8 (ESF#8), Health and Medical, ensures that information is communicated in an appropriate way, requests are logged and assigned, and missions are completed. Complex events require participation of multiple agencies. Hospitals might not be able to accomplish this using just their own resources. The current H1N1 pandemic also requires planning according to the pandemic severity index scale. As patient acuity rises and outbreaks become widespread, additional measures will need to be put into place to maintain health-care services. Continuity of operations planning (COOP) is recommended for all-hazards across the healthcare continuum. This includes hospitals, supply vendors, long-term care, private physician practices, home health agencies, and others.

Joint Hazard Vulnerability Analysis

One of the benefits of healthcare emergency response coalitions is that a dedicated meeting can be scheduled in which member hospitals can bring their facility's hazard vulnerability analysis to compare with the one that is prepared by their local and county emergency managers to ensure that it is complete and all known major hazards and priori-ties are discussed. It can then be signed off, with the date of review to document this shared task as part of Joint Commission recommendations.

Mutual Aid Support

Memorandums of understanding (MOUs) are developed as voluntary agreements by coalitions for the purpose of providing mutual aid during a disaster. The agreement ad-dresses the relationship between and among healthcare facilities and is intended to aug-ment, not replace, each facility's emergency plan. The MOU provides the framework for healthcare facilities to aid each other in emergency management through the loan of healthcare workforce personnel, pharmaceuticals, supplies and equipment, assisting with emergency evacuation, and accepting transferred patients. It also supports coordination of mutual aid with local emergency management and the health department.

Shared Protocols

When coalitions develop common protocols, it unifies the manner in which operations will occur from facility to facility. When staff agree to support other facilities during a disaster, they will already be familiar with the steps to follow. Protocols can include com-mand and control, communications, donning and doffing and decontamination, manag-ing contaminated materials, critical incident stress management, and others. Coalition training related to the protocols should be offered regularly. Facilities are encouraged to integrate the coalition protocols into their healthcare emergency plans.

Purchase of Common Equipment

Coalitions can host vendors to come in before monthly meetings to display their prod-ucts. Equipment can include communication devices, decontamination tents and supplies, personal protective equipment, evacuation equipment, and others. Members can vote on which equipment suits their common needs and get group purchase pricing. When mu-tual aid agreements are activated, personnel from other facilities will find it much easier to immediately offer support when emergency response and communications equipment is familiar to them.

Accreditation Compliance

Every year, there are new emergency management standards and recommendations for hospitals and healthcare facilities. Coalitions can sponsor accreditation updates in cooperation with their state hospital associations or expert speakers to provide updates and practical information and support the opportunity to ask questions. Best practices can be shared that might be very helpful for hospitals seeking ways of adapting their plans and procedures.

Networking

The opportunity to get to know representatives from other facilities and to share and receive information in a trusted and "safe" environment is one of the most treasured benefits for coalition members. During a disaster, when communicating with other hospitals, knowing that there is a known, recognizable person to connect with shortens the time to response as there is no need for introductions. The business at hand can be immediately attended to. Sharing facility experiences after incidents can provide psychological support as well for coalition members who might otherwise have concerns about their responses. Members have a list of facility representatives from other agencies, and they are encouraged to communicate between scheduled meetings to get any facility-specific questions answered.

Support for New and Existing Members

Turnover is expected at hospitals. Coalitions can develop HERC orientation manuals to update new members quickly and help them feel comfortable with the unique language of emergency management. When coalitions have been established for a few years, friendships can grow strong due to a level of familiarity and trust. The results of this can be observed when disasters do strike and coalition members check on each other to see if they can help out. This support can be life-saving.

Cost Savings

By offering shared training opportunities as part of coalition activities, hospitals can realize tremendous cost savings and efficiency of effort. Hospital education departments are stretched thin supporting ongoing clinical education requirements, so it makes their job much easier to support emergency management training in conjunction with others who need the same courses. Hospitals and healthcare facilities with classrooms and auditoriums can reserve space for shared trainings. Doing this fosters networking and reduces competitiveness among facilities. Coalitions have found that offering shared disaster training has also opened the door for shared nondisaster topics. Some of the disaster courses are technical in nature and just cannot be offered as online training. Cost savings for coalition members are also realized with group purchasing of equipment, including but not limited to radios, personal protective equipment, patient evacuation equipment, and patient tracking systems. One last advantage of a coalition is the assembly of a critical mass of partnerships that becomes attractive to grant sponsors who want to see cooperative work accomplished.

List at least five benefits a healthcare emergency response coalition could provide to your community.

_____

_____

_____

_____

_____

_____

_____

_____

_____

_____

_____

_____

_____

NOTE

1. U.S. Department of Homeland Security, "National Preparedness Guidelines, September 2007," Department of Homeland Security, www.dhs/gov/xlibrary/assets/National _Preparedness_ Guidelines.pdf (accessed September 30, 2009).

Existing Healthcare Emergency Response Coalition Models

CURRENT COALITION APPROACHES

A review of the current healthcare emergency response coalitions in the United States reveals that there is considerable variety in approaches. The current literature notes variation in organizational structure, membership, geographic coverage, and funding mechanisms of the existing U.S. coalitions.

The 2007 publication *Regional Approaches to Hospital Preparedness* identified and reviewed thirteen current functioning coalitions and compared and contrasted their approaches.[1] In this study, there were variations in the geographic area encompassed by the coalitions, which included city, multicity, county, multicounty, regional, state, and multistate. Funding sources to support and sustain the coalitions also varied and included municipal, county, state, and federal governmental entities. Other funding mechanisms included private foundations and coalition member dues funding, along with vendor sponsoring and sales of work products created by the coalitions.

In addition to differences in the geographic areas encompassed by the coalitions and in their funding mechanisms, variations in the fiscal agent the program resided within were noted. Coalitions were structured or incorporated within not only governmental entities (city, county, regional, and state) but also within nonprofit agencies and professional associations as well. Finally, the membership size varied considerably, with healthcare emergency coalitions having less than ten organizational members while other coalitions encompassed more than sixty member facilities.

The following list provides a diverse sampling of current healthcare emergency preparedness coalitions operating in the United States. Where available, Web links have been provided. This list is not meant to be all-inclusive but to serve as examples of coalition approaches that are functioning in communities throughout the nation.

Alabama Hospital Association Patient Transfer Systems
Alabama
www.alaha.org/

Bethesda Hospitals' Emergency Preparedness Partnership
Maryland
www.bethesda.med.navy.mil/Visitor/About_Us/Emergency_
Preparedness/

Broward County Healthcare Coalition
Florida
www.bchconline.org

Disaster Preparedness Committee of the Greater Cincinnati Health Council
Ohio
www.gchc.org/CommunityPartners/DisasterTerrorismPreparedness
Resources/tabid/180/Default.aspx

District of Columbia Emergency Healthcare Coalition
Washington, D.C.

First Coast Disaster Council of Jacksonville, Florida
Florida

Healthcare Emergency Response Association
Kentucky
www.louisvilleky.gov/Health/HERA.htm

Healthcare Emergency Response Coalition of Palm Beach County, Florida (HERC)
Florida
www.pbcms.org/HERC

Indianapolis Coalition for Patient Safety
Indiana
www.indypatientsafety.org

King County Healthcare Coalition
Washington
www.kingcounty.gov/healthservices/health/preparedness/
hccoalition.aspx

Los Angeles County Disaster Resource Centers (DRC)
California
www.cmanet.org/cme/rrr_hill.pdf

Managed Emergency Surge for Healthcare (MESH)
Indiana
www.meshcoalition.org

Metropolitan Hospital Compact
Minnesota
www.co.thurston.wa.us/HSR3/Public%20Health/Regional%20LHJ%20&%20Tribal%20MOU%20.pdf

Miami-Dade County Hospital Preparedness Consortium
Florida
www.mdchospitals.org/

New York City Hospital Emergency Preparedness Program (HEPP)
New York
www.nyc.gov/html/doh/html/bhpp/bhpp-about.shtml

Northern Virginia Hospital Alliance
Virginia
novaha.org/

Northwest Region Emergency Medical Services and Trauma Care Council
Washington
www.nwrems.org/admin/admin.htm

Regional Emergency Preparedness Steering Committee (REMPSC)
Texas
leadinghealthycommunities.com/case-studies/20010001.jsp

Rhode Island Healthcare Coalition
Rhode Island

Southwest Texas Regional Advisory Council EMS/ Hospital Disaster Group
Texas
www.strac.org/strac/committees/ehdg.shtml

As noted previously, considerable diversity exists in approaches, which suggests that there is no "best way" to develop and sustain healthcare emergency response coalitions. However, there do appear to be a number of common characteristics emerging among successful organizational collaborations. Successful healthcare emergency response coalitions have incorporated most or all of the following elements:

1. The mission, bylaws, and strategic plan are designed and executed to meet the emergency needs of both the community the coalition serves and the membership organizations that participate.

2. An all-hazards approach to disaster preparedness, response, and recovery is emphasized.

3. Geographic area and membership are clearly identified.

4. In cases in which the organizational members have a history of competitiveness and not working well together, a trusted neutral entity to sponsor the coalition can be useful during initial stages of development.

5. The coalition provides financial and other forms of incentives for hospitals and key emergency management members to participate.

6. Support of hospital executives and the leadership of the other organizational partners is secured.

7. Political support of the community stakeholders is obtained.

8. Members work year-round as a group to define gaps in planning and response, and set priorities for improvement throughout the community.

9. Early in development, the coalition develops interoperable and functional communications systems.

10. A flexible business plan is devised to ensure long-term sustainability of the coalition.

11. Federal, state, and local grants are pooled to maximize effective emergency preparedness capabilities.

12. State, regional, and local resources and assets are shared to maximize local disaster response and recovery.

13. The coalition includes other nonmembers (valued partners), which offer the coalition additional resources (examples include hospital associations, universities, and other allied health providers).

14. The coalition develops the capacity to coordinate patient transfers, as well as deployment and distribution of patient staff and supplies.

The above characteristics are strongly recommended for consideration early in the developmental stages to ensure successful coalition development.

Of the fourteen organizational characteristics listed in the text, choose at least eight that will be essential to your coalition's success. Of those selected, prioritize the order in which they will need to be accomplished.

_____

_____

_____

_____

_____

_____

_____

_____

PALM BEACH COUNTY'S HEALTHCARE EMERGENCY RESPONSE COALITION MODEL

Before Palm Beach County started a coalition, it had a history of multiagency initiatives that included the Governor's Council on Public-Private Partnerships, Safe Communities, Healthy Communities, and others. All had a mission and vision statement, a diverse group of members, and activities that supported their agendas. After Hurricane Andrew hit South Dade County in 1992, hospitals joined together to help a number of impacted hospitals, healthcare facilities, and shelters that had been damaged, lost power and water, and needed to be evacuated. Staff volunteered to work to relieve exhausted hospital personnel, transported supplies, and worked in medical tents to support primary and emergency care.

The Palm Beach County Medical Society organized a Healthcare Hurricane Preparedness Task Force. In December 2000, the Healthcare Hurricane Preparedness Task Force merged with the County Terrorism Task Force, and there was a shift away from a sole focus on tropical storms. The subsequent events associated with September 11, 2001, were felt locally. A meeting with hospitals, public health authorities, and emergency response partners was scheduled on October 4, 2001, to discuss a federal directive to plan for biological and chemical drills. There wasn't a lot of interest in the topic—until beepers started going off simultaneously around the room and one by one, people had to leave to answer them. They quickly learned about the anthrax incident at the American Media Institute building, publishers of a number of materials including the *National Enquirer*, in Boca Raton. Palm Beach County recorded the nation's first anthrax fatality as a result of a contaminated letter that had been sent to that location. There was a new awareness of how healthcare needed to work together with other emergency response agencies.

There was also a rapid realization that hospitals were not yet ready for this type of public health emergency—they did not all have the right personal protective equipment and mass decontamination equipment, and they needed training on how to use it. Palm Healthcare Foundation rose to the challenge with a $250,000 grant for an initial purchase of communications equipment, hazardous materials suits, and mobile decontamination units for the thirteen hospitals within Palm Beach County. A decision was made to merge the County Terrorism Task Force with the Palm Beach Medical Society's Emergency Medical Services Disaster Preparedness Committee. A nationally recognized consultant, Craig DeAtley, PA-C, was asked to facilitate the development of initial common protocols that the hospitals could integrate with their planning.

Support for the hospitals from emergency response partners such as the Palm Beach County Department of Health, Palm Beach County Emergency Management, Palm Beach County Fire Rescue, the Palm Beach County Sheriff's Office, and the Palm Beach County Health Care District led to a second grant award from Palm Healthcare Foundation for the development of a model plan and eventually resulted in the formal development of the structure known as the Healthcare Emergency Response Coalition of Palm Beach County (HERC). There was immediate recognition that there needed to be overall interoperability, including common communication systems, joint training, shared protocols, and memorandums of understanding for mutual aid.

One of the more dramatic early milestones for HERC occurred when the CEOs of all thirteen hospitals in the county signed a common memorandum of understanding to support the coalition and to share staff, supplies, and bed space as needed in a disaster. This coincided with the development of a formal mission, vision, and operating guidelines for the coalition; elections of leaders; a steering committee; and subcommittees. Membership was formalized and eventually grew to include twenty-two agencies.

HERC Member Organizations	**Regional Health and Medical Representatives**
Acute care hospitals	American Red Cross
Specialty hospitals	School health program
Mental health centers	Special needs shelters
Long-term care alliance	Healthcare foundation
Crisis consortium	County public health (ESF-8 and Epi)
Municipal and county law enforcement	Healthcare district
EMS and fire rescue	Hospital and healthcare association
Dialysis coalition and renal associates	Local universities
Blood centers	Medical reserve corps
Veterinarian agency	
Local emergency management	

Acute care hospitals included private and public nonprofit community hospitals, for-profit hospitals, corporate network hospitals, and the Veterans Administration Medical Center that was within the county. Prior to HERC, the hospitals tended to be competitive in nature and not eager to share any information about their emergency plans, activities, training needs, or on-hand supplies. Capacities and capabilities were not fully understood, and even if hospitals needed help, many of them would not have known whom to contact or how to access resources. The culture completely changed within a couple of years to one of being supportive to other member hospitals and being much more open about sharing information.

The CEOs of each hospital were asked to name one designated and two alternate representatives each year. The concept of "three-deep" is rooted in incident command system principles, essentially ensuring that there would always be a person available to attend the meetings. HERC specified that one of the assigned hospital representatives should be an infection control preventionist (ICP). This supported participation in a syndromic surveillance committee and using a syndromic surveillance system in the hospitals to be used as an early warning for outbreaks or incidents. The hospital representatives were from a range of departments including emergency preparedness, safety and security, emergency, risk management, education, and administration. This offered subject matter expertise when specific issues were brought up, new standards emerged, or incidents occurred like security threats or hospital fires.

Every year gave an opportunity to recognize and review the achievements of the past twelve months, rotate officers, and document events, exercises, training, and special achievements. This summary took the shape of an annual HERC community summary report, which was released back to all participating agencies, county and state partners, and other interested parties, including other states who were interested in forming their own coalitions. An annual recognition dinner is held to honor officers for their service and those who were outstanding in leading committees, special projects, or support to HERC membership. For example, fire rescue was given an award for assisting with training of hospital staff in operations level and decontamination.

List stakeholders from your community who will be needed for your HERC to be successful.

_____

_____

_____

_____

_____

_____

_____

_____

_____

_____

_____

_____

PALM BEACH COUNTY'S INCENTIVES FOR HERC MEMBERSHIP

Common Communication Mechanisms and Interoperability

The coalition supported the initial purchase of 800-MHz radios that were programmed for interoperability by local emergency management at no cost to the hospitals. A "hospital common channel" was identified for alert purposes, and all hospitals were given a matrix for reaching each other and emergency response partners. Communications training was included at one of the meetings by a county communications subject matter expert, to ensure that members knew how to operate the radios. Weekly roll calls were initiated and results were documented and shared back to members, who used the feedback to include with their Joint Commission paperwork for communication interoperability.

Communications were enhanced for the coalition with event management software to be primarily used by the hospitals for internal use, but which also allowed for external transfer of information to the county emergency operations center (EOC). Hospital command center 24/7 contact information was shared with the EOC, in addition to a 24/7 contact list for HERC membership. Access information was given to all members to get signed up and approved for threat notification from law enforcement and for epidemiologic alerts and reports from the health department. Communications also included e-mail distribution lists that reminded membership of upcoming meetings with agendas, review of meeting minutes, and training opportunities. A website was established for HERC at www.pbcms.org/herc, which includes password protection, to access documents, upcoming exercise opportunities, a training calendar with direct links to registration, resource information related to activation, emergency contacts for county public health, and links to federal, state, and local disaster response agencies.

Shared Training Opportunities

The cost for hiring a consultant to conduct emergency preparedness training for your hospital can run approximately $1,500 to $3,000 per class. Unfortunately, attendance can be low due to department staffing needs, and multiple class sessions are just not cost effective. A hospital coalition that uses shared training opportunities increases the number of students attending from the pool of hospitals and also maintains consistency of what is taught in the curriculum. Coalitions can cut their costs by requesting training support from local emergency management, fire rescue, regional trainers, or university disaster-trained staff. Hospitals with large classrooms and auditoriums can be rotated so that travel times to various geographic locations are equitably distributed. There is no cost to use county facilities such as agricultural extension offices, parks and recreation, emergency operations center, public safety institutes, and others with training classrooms.

Joint Exercises

Hospitals can choose to exercise independently and also participate in community-wide, county, regional, state, and federal exercises. This fulfills Joint Commission accreditation requirements and makes the planning end of exercises easier. Local emergency management wants hospitals and healthcare agencies to exercise with them, and they are supportive of hospitals adding objectives that they want to test in addition to those listed as part of the exercise. When cooperating with local and regional planners, there is the advantage that the exercises will be rotated based on prioritization of a threat or the perception of a need to refresh skills for a particular type of incident. In South Florida, the exercises are rotated to include themes like "Mass Migration," "Cruise Ship Bio Outbreak," "Super Bowl Chemical Release," "Radiological Dirty Bomb," "Protestor Threats," and others. Hospital coalition members volunteer to be included with the exercise design team and help with the planning, enlisting partner agencies to participate in the exercise, and ensuring that the after-action review process is completed for the coalition group and as part of the larger group. All exercises are Homeland Security Exercise Evaluation Program (HSEEP) compliant, with defined target capabilities to be exercised and documentation of the entire process from planning through corrective action reports. Coalition members that participate in the exercises receive copies of the after-action reviews to include with their documentation and to use to improve planning at their own facilities.

Mutual Aid

HERC, like other coalitions, completed an MOU between its members. It is one thing to have an MOU that agrees to support a process to share staff, supplies, and bed space; it is quite another thing to witness how an MOU can be used. During the major hurricanes that hit Florida in 2004–2005, the experience was intense, with sustained power outages, fuel shortages, supply limitations, martial law, curfews, and hospitals experiencing a surge of patients that included persons with special needs, chronic disease exacerbations, carbon monoxide poisoning, and injuries. Coalition hospitals helped each other out with distribution of patients and sharing supplies, which included items as simple as extra batteries for the mobile radios or as complex as generators. Being able to call a HERC contact within another facility and immediately work through issues was effective. One hospital called in that their backup generator was failing. Another hospital responded with the answer "What size do you need?" and then "I have a spare and it's on its way to you."

The hurricanes made everyone realize how many power-dependent patients are living in communities, who require dialysis, oxygen and nebulizer support, ventilators, power chairs, morphine pumps, and other equipment. Mitigation measures were put into place as part of the after-action review process to reduce vulnerabilities for when such a power outage would occur again, and it did. Every incident is unique and affords an opportunity to learn from it and become stronger and more resilient.

Hurricane Wilma in October 2005 resulted in eighty hospitals losing power and being maintained on backup generators. Some lost water pressure. Physician practices lost power and communication capabilities, and some had physical damage as well. Community pharmacies were closed, as they did not have backup generators. The need for primary care services was evident, with hospitals being surged with patients who did not need high-level care but there was not another alternate in place for them. All of these situations were included in after-action reporting, with measures now put into place so there will be less of an impact when it occurs again. HERC now has a relationship with the Medical Reserve Corps, a pre-registered and pre-credentialed supplemental healthcare workforce. They are included in HERC joint training and exercises, which adds to the capabilities of an overall response network.

Purchasing Power

HERC receives monthly sponsorship support from a range of vendors who are selected to give a three-minute overview of their products to members and have a display for members to visit before and after the meetings. Because of the number of agencies represented, group rate purchase prices are extended to coalition members. Vendors can be invited to participate in exercises to evaluate various types of equipment. For example, during an emergency evacuation drill, products can be reviewed that include patient evacuation equipment and patient tracking devices.

Vendors are available to guide use of the products. When equipment is chosen for a group purchase for all of the hospitals, it increases the comfort level of staff who respond to help during a disaster as part of mutual aid support and are familiar with the devices, as they are used also at their facility.

Other benefits that HERC members have expressed include:

- Assistance with disaster-related grant submission/compliance to complete deliverables
- Active participation and input into county, regional, and state emergency management planning
- Real-time situational awareness of emergency threats in their area
- A unified voice in regional and state decision-making processes
- Enhanced and redundant communication capabilities with emergency management and other key members and partners
- The ability to draw staff, supplies, and equipment from other members during disasters
- Timely access to county health and medical assets during disasters
- Enhanced member preparedness and response and recovery capabilities
- Improved member organization abilities to communicate and work collaboratively with each other and with county, regional, and state agencies
- A nonemergency resource network to assist in meeting day-to-day operational needs
- Relationship building with staff from other hospitals, healthcare providers, fire rescue, police, EMS, health department, school health personnel, and others
- Improved overall facility capabilities to respond to all-hazard events

EVALUATION OF THE EFFECTIVENESS OF HERC

There are tangible and intangible indicators for how HERC is effective. Tangible indicators include:

- 100 percent participation by hospitals in the coalition
- Performance of weekly roll calls as an indicator for communication interoperability readiness
- Attendance levels at training across hospitals and healthcare facilities to maintain individual and collective emergency response teams
- Attendance levels at meetings per sign-in sheets to receive information updates
- Participation levels in joint exercises and drills
- Number of hospitals participating in syndromic surveillance
- Number of hospitals enrolled in situational awareness notification systems
- Equipment inventories for personal protective equipment, radiation detection, mass decontamination capability, and mass casualty supplies
- Common all-hazard protocols
- Consistent standards for disaster burn care
- Recognition from national-level agencies such as the CDC, the AMA's Model Community Program, and NACCHO's Best Practice award

Intangible benefits for coalition members include:

- Emotional support during disasters ("We're in this together and we'll get through it")
- Networking opportunities
- Feeling that they have active participation in local, county, regional, and state planning
- Inclusion of health and medical issues within all other emergency management planning

List five benefits that are priorities for a coalition to be considered successful.

_____

_____

_____

_____

_____

_____

_____

_____

_____

_____

_____

_____

_____

_____

NOTE

1. B. Maldin, C. Lam, C. Franco, D. Press, R. Waldhorn, E. Toner, T. O'Toole, and T. V. Inglesby, *Regional Approaches to Hospital Preparedness* (Baltimore: Center for Biosecurity of the University of Pittsburgh Medical Center, 2007).

4

How to Structure a Healthcare Emergency Response Coalition

INITIAL STEPS

The structure of a healthcare coalition is important. There are several items that need to be addressed early in the planning process to enable the coalition to maximize its effectiveness. The initial steps center on identifying the structural makeup of the coalition. One of the first items that should be addressed is identifying which stakeholders need to participate in the coalition. Based on those stakeholders, the coalition should prioritize gaining support from the leadership within each member organization. Next, the ideal makeup of the types of professions within an organization should be established. In addition, financial matters should be decided with respect to what organization will serve as a fiscal agent for the coalition to handle any financial administrative issues that arise.

Bringing Key Stakeholders Together

As discussed in Chapter 1, coalitions typically start when a small group of individuals comes together to address an issue that none of the individuals are in a position to address by themselves. This small group is tasked with identifying and bringing together the other stakeholders that are needed within the coalition. If the initial group identifies a problem that impacts their organization and they decide that a coalition is the best way to address the issue, they should begin by contacting similar organizations in their region that face the same challenge and inviting them to join the coalition. For example, if a small group of hospitals identifies that patient surge capacity is a concern for their hospital, they should invite the other hospitals in the region who not only would face the same surge capacity issue, but who in combination could effectively design a regional solution to the problem.

As the early coalition members identify other organizations to invite to join the coalition, every effort should be made to include all organizations that have a similar function. In the hospital example above, all hospitals in a region need to participate. If one hospital seems reluctant, they should continue to be invited and be provided with information on the activities of the coalition in hopes of attracting them at a future date.

After the coalition establishes the healthcare stakeholders who will be members, the next step is identifying the emergency preparedness organizations that will be a part of the coalition. The emergency preparedness organizations will be the critical link to a community's overall response planning, ensuring that the healthcare community is included in the overall system response and planning. These organizations are similar across most jurisdictions. They include law enforcement, fire rescue, emergency management, public health, and any healthcare government systems or taxing districts.

The emergency preparedness community brings a level of expertise and discipline to the table that is outside the scope of most healthcare professions. Law enforcement and fire rescue operate in a world of unified incident command to manage the crises they face on a regular basis. Emergency management and public health live in this world as well, as they bring their expertise and coordination to large-scale natural and man-made disaster events. A healthcare coalition enables hospitals, physicians, and other healthcare providers to be trained in crisis management protocols so they can work hand in hand off the same playbook with their emergency preparedness partners. The initial step of identifying and inviting the healthcare and emergency preparedness stakeholders begins to lay the foundation for how the coalition will structure itself.

Once the initial core group of stakeholders has been identified, the ancillary or extended healthcare organizations should be included as well. Referring to the hospital example, the next healthcare group to invite to the coalition might involve the nursing homes operating in the region. At this point, a decision should be made as to whether all nursing homes will be extended the opportunity to be members of the coalition or if a single representative from the nursing home community should be invited, who can function as a liaison back to all the nursing homes in the region. This process should continue within other healthcare disciplines including physicians, pharmacies, dialysis providers, urgent care clinics, and other healthcare providers, until the group feels that all members of the healthcare community required to make the coalition effective have been identified.

In Chapter 3 you identified a list of stakeholders from your community who will be needed for the coalition to be successful. Now, identify the appropriate stakeholder level of participation for your coalition (e.g., Will all nursing homes be members or will there be just a single liaison member from the nursing home community or local association?)

_____

_____

_____

_____

_____

_____

_____

_____

_____

_____

_____

Enlisting Support of CEOs

After the list of stakeholders is identified, the organizations must be approached and invited to join the coalition. Since the magnitude of the challenge the coalition is being established to address is significant, the CEO or director of the organization or agency should be approached. Buy-in and support from the top is the best way to ensure long-term commitments from organizations. CEOs should be invited to initial meetings to help explain how the coalition will function and the types of activities it will work on.

Inviting the group of CEOs to an introductory educational meeting can serve as an effective venue to enlist support. During this event, or as a separate stand-alone event, a tabletop exercise that addresses key challenges the coalition will be working on can be a very effective way to enlighten CEOs on the issues faced in the community. For example, if hospital evacuation is a potential issue for hospitals located in areas where hurricanes and tropical storms occur, a tabletop exercise with the CEOs that presents the challenges that will be faced can provide real-world scenarios that demonstrate the need for the coalition's activities.

Recognition opportunities can also serve as positive reinforcement when trying to enlist the support of the organization and agency CEOs. Recognition lunches thanking the CEOs for their commitment to the coalition can be an effective way to foster support from the CEOs and instill the view that the coalition efforts are worth the time and commitment of the organization. Thank-you letters, announcements when new hospitals or agencies join the coalition, and general updates on coalition activities can serve as simple and inexpensive ways to keep the CEOs engaged and up-to-date.

Make a list of the CEOs from each of the organizations that will be invited to join the coalition, including all of their contact information.

_____

_____

_____

_____

_____

_____

_____

_____

_____

_____

_____

_____

_____

Designating the Organization's Representatives

Once CEOs have been identified and invited to have their organization join the coalition, they should then be given the opportunity to designate staff to the coalition on their behalf. Guidance can be provided to the CEOs in identifying the types of staff who would be most valuable to the coalition. For example, if the organization is a hospital, the infection control practitioner, emergency department director, and safety officer all represent skill sets that would bring value to the coalition. In some cases, a hospital CEO may find it beneficial to have their COO or another administrator involved. This is a decision that should ultimately be made by each CEO. However, recommendations or suggestions from the coalition are a good idea to help foster the skill sets needed by the coalition and to offer the CEO ideas for who on their staff would be the most appropriate designee. As discussed in Chapter 3, the Palm Beach County HERC utilizes a designated representative from each organization and two alternate designees. The backup representatives ensure that the absence of another does not slow down any activities and also brings additional perspectives to the coalition.

The agencies will also need to designate a representative. Fire rescue and law enforcement will likely already have an emergency management designee who would bring value to the coalition. In addition, the public health department would also have someone in a position related to emergency preparedness who would be a strong designee to the coalition. Within all organizations, someone usually has specific responsibilities during disaster events. Individuals who will be responding to and working through disasters are the individuals whom the coalition should target.

Indicate the disciplines that the coalition will target for membership from each potential member.

_____

_____

_____

_____

_____

_____

_____

_____

_____

_____

_____

_____

_____

Merits of the Coalition Structure

The structure of the group can take several forms. This book advocates the coalition framework as a flexible and nonthreatening approach. Other frameworks include partnerships, associations, affiliations, and other more formal, semilegal structures. The more formal structures bring with them potential barriers to effective implementation. For example, for-profit hospital chains may be reluctant to enter into legal arrangements with competing hospitals. Formal arrangements often include some type of legal contract that binds the activities of the partner entities to an agreement or contract. In some cases, this may be tied to federal or state grant funding such that all parties receiving financing are tied to the requirements of the grant. If the formal arrangement brings commitments that for-profit and private, nonprofit organizations do not want to adhere to, then the structure itself may struggle to attract the needed members to the group.

The coalition structure outlined in this book is less formal and less threatening to the proprietary needs of many for-profit and private, nonprofit organizations. The coalition structure can include structural frameworks defined through bylaws, operating guidelines, policies and procedures, and other vehicles that do not contractually bind an organization. In the Palm Beach County HERC experience, the coalition made the decision to utilize operating guidelines to facilitate the activities of the coalition. The operating guidelines outlined the committee and officer structure, quorum, meeting schedules and procedures, member organizations, designated representatives, and other structural mechanisms that allow the coalition to function effectively. Sample operating guidelines are included in Appendix C.

This approach proved to be attractive to a coalition comprising four different for-profit hospital chains, three independent nonprofit hospitals, one public hospital, a VA hospital, and a state tuberculosis hospital.

The coalition structure utilized in Palm Beach County's HERC also positioned the group to receive grants in a noncompetitive environment. Each coalition member, including both hospitals and agencies, was able to independently pursue and receive grants to fund emergency preparedness planning, equipment, technology, and funding for exercises and drills, as well as to participate in community-wide grants from foundations, state, and federal sources. The dual approach that the coalition structure allowed has enabled the community to maximize the resources available for emergency preparedness. Other coalitions have utilized a slightly more formal structure in the form of bylaws. Bylaws tend to be documents of a defined legal entity.

Fiscal Agent

Early in the planning stage, the coalition should designate a fiscal agent. A fiscal agent can be almost any legal organization, like a business or agency. A fiscal agent is needed for the coalition because state, federal, and foundation grantors require a legal entity to receive funding. Without a fiscal agent, a coalition would likely be unable to apply for funding, fully benefit from group purchasing, and reconcile financial matters. Fiscal agents typically will charge a small percentage for administering the financial dealings of the coalition. The fiscal agent can receive funds from grants, membership dues, donations, and revenues if the coalition sells any goods or services. In addition, the fiscal agent can facilitate the purchase of any goods or services needed by the coalition.

List five reasons the coalition structure could support the desired goals of the group and at least five challenges that will be faced.

_____

_____

_____

_____

_____

_____

_____

_____

_____

_____

_____

_____

_____

_____

Selection of a fiscal agent should be done with great care. Since the fiscal agent will handle all financial matters, the coalition should choose a stable, reliable, and trustworthy organization. In addition, the organization should be one that will remain impartial and not hinder the activities of the coalition.

In Palm Beach County, HERC designated the Palm Beach County Medical Society Services to serve as the fiscal agent. The Medical Society Services is a nonprofit 501(c)(3) corporation. Designating the Medical Society to serve as the fiscal agent gave the coalition a legal organization from which to apply for grants, conduct group purchasing, engage consultants, and to have someone account for the finances of the coalition.

Several positive outcomes resulted from utilizing the Medical Society Services for the fiscal agent role. The Medical Society had a relationship with Palm Healthcare Foundation that facilitated the first grant funding to purchase communication radios and personal protective equipment for the hospitals. The Medical Society was viewed as a neutral party, so there was a level of trust that the funding would be distributed fairly to all organizations. In addition, the neutrality of the Medical Society never caused any of the competing hospitals to have concerns that a competitive advantage was being gained as a result of planning and sharing information together. Had another hospital been chosen to serve as the fiscal agent, the loss of impartiality garnered through the Medical Society might have derailed some of the coalition's activities.

As Palm Beach County's HERC evolved, the Medical Society was increasingly viewed in a positive light by the hospital, agencies, and emergency preparedness community for the very important role it played as the HERC fiscal agent.

Develop a list of the potential organizations that can serve as a fiscal agent for the coalition. Include the pros and cons for each organization.

_____

_____

_____

_____

_____

_____

_____

_____

_____

_____

_____

_____

_____

LEADERSHIP QUALITIES FOR THE CHAIRPERSON

Choosing a chairperson for a coalition is an important task. The role encompasses strategic planning, assessment and reassessment of achieving goals, developing agendas for both the steering committee and the general membership meetings, facilitating discussions, and serving as the voice of the coalition to represent the healthcare mission within emergency response.

Considerations for whom to nominate for the position include:

- A member of the healthcare community, preferably from an accredited hospital
- Familiarity with hospital and healthcare regulatory standards, including state and federal guidance
- Experience being actively involved with hospital and community disaster planning and response, preferably with experience serving in a role within his or her own hospital's incident command system structure
- Good communication skills
- Solid computer skills including fluency with e-mail, scheduling of meetings, document development, and basic spreadsheet analysis
- Development of training materials for professional and public education programs
- Experience in successful delivery of presentations
- Training in disaster awareness, operations-level disaster courses, disaster behavioral health, risk communications, continuity of operations planning (COOP), hospital incident command system (HICS)

- Certification in national incident management system (NIMS) courses, including a minimum of IS-100, IS-200, IS-300, IS-400, IS-700, and IS-800
- Certification in the Homeland Security Exercise and Evaluation Program (HSEEP)
- Experience with grant writing and grant management

Additional leadership qualities that are needed for the role include:

- Professionalism—someone who has the dedication and sense of purpose to accomplish advancement in healthcare emergency preparedness levels for the coalition and who can serve as a role model to foster a culture of accountability for the responsibilities associated with the continuous cycle of preparedness, response, and recovery
- Team-building capabilities—the ability to remain neutral and work collaboratively with a diverse group of members, encouraging people to become engaged, to remain focused, and to understand the significance of his or her work for the coalition
- A positive attitude, outgoing personality, and a calm demeanor

---

List at least five leadership qualities your coalition chairperson will need.

_____

_____

_____

_____

_____

_____

_____

_____

_____

_____

_____

_____

_____

_____

ADMINISTRATIVE ACTIVITIES AND STRUCTURE

Naming and Branding the Coalition

Naming and branding the coalition as a unique entity may appear straightforward, but time and thought need to be given to it. The name chosen for the coalition should have at least two primary characteristics: first, the name of the coalition ideally indicates the function or purpose of the coalition; and second, the name identifies the geographic area in which the coalition operates. Often the coalition's geographic coverage area can be defined by political boundaries such as city, county, region, or state. This was the case with the Healthcare Emergency Response Coalition (HERC) of Palm Beach County, Florida, where both the geographic area and the function of the coalition were incorporated into the name.

Branding the coalition serves an important function, just like the name chosen. Foremost, effective branding of the coalition name ensures the identify of the coalition as a unique centralizing entity, in which its members, governmental agencies, community stakeholders, potential funders, and the community at large view the coalition as a major health and medical coordinating force in preparedness for, response to, and recovery from disaster events. Branding can be reinforced not only with an appropriate name but with congruent logo, stationery, annual community reports, and a website. This was the case in Palm Beach County, Florida, with HERC. Within two years of its inception, HERC (which represented all fifteen hospitals as well as the key health and emergency community partners) was acknowledged in the county, region, and state as an essential local health and medical emergency planning and coordinating force.

Write at least three possible names for your coalition and list at least four branding methods that might be used to promote the coalition's visibility in the health and emergency management community.

_____

_____

_____

_____

_____

_____

_____

_____

_____

_____

_____

_____

_____

Mission Statement and Purpose(s)

A mission statement is a short statement that captures the purpose of an organization. The mission statement should serve to guide the actions of the organization, identifying its goals and providing a sense of direction for the organization.

A purpose statement is a declarative sentence that summarizes the broad goal of an organization. Purpose statements can be included in a strategic plan to provide a broader description of what an organization (or in this case, a coalition) intends to pursue. To be effective, purpose statements should be:

- Complementary to the mission statement
- Concise, limited to one or two sentences
- Goal-oriented

Defining the mission and purpose(s) may also appear straightforward, but considerable time and thought need to be given during this stage of development. Development of a mission and purpose often takes considerable negotiations among the members in reaching consensus. However, the time and effort in development of an agreed-upon mission and purpose will prove time well spent to facilitate and simplify the coalition's strategic planning process and other development stages that will follow. A sample of a mission statement and purposes are provided here for consideration.

HERC MISSION

To develop and promote the healthcare emergency preparedness, response and recovery capabilities of Palm Beach County, Florida

HERC PURPOSES

- To provide a forum for the healthcare community to interact with one another and other response agencies at a county, regional, and state level to promote emergency preparedness
- To coordinate and improve the delivery of healthcare emergency response services in collaboration with other stakeholders
- To foster communication between local, regional, and state entities on community-wide emergency planning, response, and recovery
- To ensure overall readiness through coordination of community-wide training and exercises
- To promote preparedness in the healthcare community through standardized practices and integration with other response partners

Draft an initial mission statement and state at least three purposes for your coalition.

_____

_____

_____

_____

_____

_____

_____

_____

_____

_____

_____

_____

_____

_____

_____

Operating Procedures (Bylaws)

It is critical that all members agree to follow established operating procedures or guidelines. Depending on the organizational structure, these guidelines may be referred to as "coalition bylaws" or "standard operating procedures" (SOP). Coalition bylaws often incorporate at a minimum the following elements:

- Name of the coalition
- Mission statement
- Purpose(s)
- Composition and types of organizational membership ("members" versus "partners"; voting versus nonvoting participants)
- Designated and alternate representatives
- Terms and confirmation of representatives
- Frequency and types of established meetings
- Committee structure
- Quorum and voting procedures
- Parliamentary procedures and decision-making process
- Fiscal agent and financial procedures
- Officers and committee structure
- Administrative staff support

The operating procedures and related policies and procedures should be reviewed for modifications annually by the membership. During the formation of the coalition, do not underestimate the time required to complete this task. Considerable give and take and compromise is essential as the members define their roles and relationships. An example of operating guidelines (bylaws) is found in Appendix C. As with all sample documents provided in this guidebook, modification and customization to meet the specific needs of the community and coalition membership is essential.

Briefly describe the process that will be utilized in the development of the bylaws. Will a committee be assigned this task? Who should be represented on this committee? Will a consultant or neutral party be needed to assist in this task? List at least eight basic elements that your coalition will need to delineate in its bylaws.

_____

_____

_____

_____

_____

_____

_____

_____

_____

_____

_____

_____

_____

_____

Mutual Aid: Memorandum of Understanding (MOU)

This document provides the key elements during a disaster upon which the member organizations agree to work together in assisting one another. Moreover, this document addresses the relationships between and among healthcare facilities and is intended to augment, not replace, a facility's emergency management/disaster plan. The mutual aid agreement also provides the framework for healthcare facilities to coordinate as a single healthcare facility mutual aid system (HFMAS) in coordination with the county emergency management, health department, and municipal and private sectors during disaster planning and response. This document does not replace but rather supplements the rules and procedures governing interaction with other organizations during a disaster.

Specifically, the agreement is for participating healthcare facilities to aid one another in their emergency management by authorizing the loan/utilization of medical personnel, pharmaceuticals, supplies, equipment, or assistance with emergency healthcare facility evacuation and patient transfers. The agreement should be signed by each member organization's top leadership prior to agreeing to coalition membership.

Key elements that should be delineated in the mutual aid memorandum of understanding are:

- Document name and parties entering in the agreement
- Introduction and background
- Purpose of the mutual aid MOU
- Definition of terms
- General principles of understanding
- Specific principles of understanding
- Transfer of pharmaceuticals, supplies, and equipment
- Transfer/evacuation of patients
- Communication methodology
- Miscellaneous provisions (term of agreement, confidentiality, insurance, liability)

An example of a mutual aid memorandum of understanding from the Palm Beach County HERC is provided in Appendix B.

Briefly describe the process that will be utilized in developing the mutual aid agreement. Will a committee be assigned this task? Who should be represented on this committee? Will a consultant be needed to assist in this task?

_____

_____

_____

_____

_____

_____

_____

_____

_____

_____

_____

_____

Establishing Committees and Organizational Structure

The steering committee is the executive body of the coalition. It consists of representative hospitals, agencies, and other responders with complementary emergency response roles. The steering committee is responsible for oversight of operations and coordination of coalition activities, setting agendas, running meetings, making policy recommendations to the general membership, and overseeing the numerous administrative functions of the coalition.

Officers should be elected within twelve months of the formation of the group, and at a minimum should include a chair, vice-chair, treasurer, and secretary. In addition to their regular duties, the officers represent the coalition at local, state, regional, and national meetings and conferences.

In addition to a steering committee, the coalition should consider additional subcommittees. Subcommittees assist with executing the key purposes and related activities of the coalition. These committees are responsible for researching, developing plans, and executing the decisions of the general membership. A committee is often chaired by a steering committee member and includes at least three general member representatives. The committees meet regularly and report activities to the steering committee and general membership at the monthly meetings. In the Palm Beach County HERC, four standing subcommittees were formed:

- Education/training committee
- Communication committee
- Syndromic surveillance and patient tracking committee
- Public affairs and sustainability committee

One or more ad hoc or temporary task forces/committees may be formed from time to time to address a special issue or task that does not warrant a long-term standing committee. In these cases, an ad hoc task force consisting of several members appointed from the coalition membership may be formed. The task force should be charged with a very clear role to ensure effectiveness. Upon completion of the ad hoc committee's duties, it is dissolved. For a full description of the roles and functions of coalition committees, refer to the sample operational guidelines provided in Appendix C.

Following the development of operational procedures or bylaws, it is important to clarify the coalition's structure by utilizing an organizational chart. The organizational chart will assist members and other community leaders to better understand how the coalition operates and the role each partner plays.

Meetings, Minutes, Location, and Administrative Support

It is recommended that professional guidelines be established for meetings and clearly specified in the coalition's written operational procedures. Other suggestions include:

- Schedule meetings well in advance.
- Prepare and adhere to agendas.
- Take and distribute formal minutes.
- Conduct meetings in an orderly fashion according to established rules, such as Robert's Rules of Order.

Which organizational members will be represented on the steering committee? What standing committees will be needed? What officers will be needed? What organization(s) could be the sponsoring or fiscal agent, or will the coalition establish an independent nonprofit 501(c)(3)?

_____

_____

_____

_____

_____

_____

_____

_____

_____

_____

_____

_____

Location for the meeting is important as well. A neutral location can often serve in promoting an egalitarian atmosphere for the smaller member organizations. Other considerations in choosing a location include

- Adequate room size
- Geographic distance from member facilities
- Cost
- Availability

Communications

Much of the communications between formal coalition meetings, during nonemergency periods, can be accomplished by utilizing e-mail. Other methods of regular information sharing include:

- Timely distribution of formal meeting minutes via e-mail and posting on a secure website
- Coalition website with a password/secured section for coalition members only
- Weekly or monthly e-mail update reports by coalition officers
- Regular distribution of member contact information, including at a minimum member representatives' phone number and e-mail address

- Training opportunities available for members placed on coalition website calendar and e-mailed to representatives
- Newsletters quarterly (via Web and/or print)
- Annual coalition progress report for members and community stakeholders
- Annual coalition recognition dinner

List at least five methods of communication that might be utilized by your coalition with the membership and community stakeholders.

_____

_____

_____

_____

_____

_____

_____

_____

_____

_____

_____

_____

_____

5

Establishing Goals, Implementing Objectives, and Developing Emergency Response Procedures

Some of the most important elements in the development of a healthcare emergency response coalition are the establishment of coalition goals, implementing objectives, and developing standardized emergency response procedures. The goals and objectives will outline and direct the coalition's activities into the future. This is the point in the development process when the key stakeholders will identify what activities need to take place to address the community challenges that initially led to the establishment of the coalition. This process will include the development of the standardized emergency response procedures that will guide the coalition members in a standardized approach to an all-hazards response protocol.

This chapter will walk through some very critical processes to set the coalition on the path to success. What follows is a discussion of the strategic planning process and some of the basic steps that can be utilized to develop a strategic plan, a section on implementing objectives, and a section on the development of standardized emergency response procedures.

STRATEGIC PLANNING
Strategic planning serves as an organized process to identify needs, assess gaps, and develop objectives and action items to accomplish the goals of the coalition. Strategic planning can include many steps. Some of the basic components include the development of a mission statement and purpose statements, a SWOT analysis, goals and objectives, and action-item implementing steps. The following sections review some of the basic steps and provide examples that can be utilized to help form a coalition's strategic plan. In addition, a sample strategic plan is included in Appendix D.

Facilitator
Before the strategic planning process begins, a facilitator should be selected to guide the group. Secure an objective, neutral, outside facilitator with national disaster response experience and knowledge and experience in the local community if possible. Emergency management within a region can serve as a good source for finding a facilitator if there are no obvious choices. Also, check around with other coalition members and other coalitions throughout the United States. Very capable facilitators are available. Keep in mind that

there will be costs associated with the facilitator. Costs will vary based on the scope of work and the number of days the strategic planning process will span. Budget appropriately!

The facilitator's responsibilities will depend on the scope of the engagement. Possible facilitator responsibilities may include:

- Guiding the group through the development of a mission statement, SWOT analysis, and identification of goals, objectives, and action items
- Providing standardized training materials
- Developing, coordinating, and evaluating a regional exercise
- Researching and developing recommendations related to the purchasing of personal protective equipment (Hazmat and other associated equipment)
- Recommending protocols to address regulatory issues
- Serving as a clearinghouse for training resources

List potential facilitators for your coalition's strategic planning process. List potential deliverables you would like the facilitator to execute during the strategic planning process.

_____

_____

_____

_____

_____

_____

_____

_____

_____

_____

_____

_____

_____

SWOT Analysis

SWOT analysis is a powerful strategic planning technique for understanding the strengths and weaknesses of an organization and for looking at the opportunities and threats it faces. What makes SWOT particularly powerful is that, with a little thought, it can help uncover opportunities that the coalition is well poised to take advantage of and help understand weaknesses and threats facing the coalition that might otherwise have gone unnoticed. What follows is an example of a SWOT analysis that could apply to a healthcare emergency response coalition.

Strengths
- Funding source: foundation
- Multidisciplinary composition: public health, fire rescue, public safety
- Hospital perspective
- Motivated to succeed
- Technical support
- Different specialty perspectives
- Realistic fear of unknown
- Using the work that has been completed to date
- Embracing all response participants

Weaknesses
- Inconsistent funding
- Time constraints of participants—being involved, being productive
- Varying commitments
- No full-time person
- Overwhelming information demands
- Missing potential partners
- Need to share vision, get the word out (everyone doesn't know us)
- Need more focus

Opportunities
- Funding
- To be a model program
- Improve profile with public
- To do something concrete—demonstrable
- More inclusion by others, like emergency management, CEMP, CERT, etc.
- More exposure and interaction with elected officials and the state
- Affiliate with a university—brings national expertise to the table
- Expanded cross-training with law enforcement (internal and external)
- Increase best practices model contributions
- Use our power in political arena (sphere of influence)
- Real-event success

Threats
- Lack of focus—chasing too many opportunities
- Politics becoming divisive among members
- Complacency and stagnation
- Better mousetrap—someone else gets to Joint Commission first
- External competition
- Perceived or actual failure during a real event
- Loss or reduction of internal support from organization CEOs and directors

Review the description of the SWOT analysis in the text. Complete a SWOT analysis for your coalition using the space below.

Strengths	Weaknesses
Opportunities	**Threats**

Goals and Objectives

After establishing mission and purpose statements and conducting a SWOT analysis, the coalition should develop goals and objectives for the upcoming year(s). One-year, two-year, and five-year goals and objectives are not uncommon in a strategic plan. However, for a new coalition, establishing yearly goals and objectives provides an opportunity for the coalition to more quickly address items and develop a sense of accomplishment to build on. The number of goals and objectives should be between three and seven, with each being attainable within the specified time period. A common error in establishing goals during strategic planning is to set unattainable goals or to set too many goals for the coalition to reasonably be expected to accomplish. What follows are some example goals for a healthcare emergency response coalition:

- Stay true to the mission and purpose.
- Make needed revisions to the operating guidelines.
- Make needed revisions to the standardized emergency response procedures.
- Ensure timely and effective communication between HERC members, the fiscal agent, member CEOs, elected officials, and the public.
- Develop new standardized emergency response procedures for situations that currently have no procedures (e.g., medical surge, fatality management, patient tracking, syndromic surveillance, behavioral and mental health recovery).
- Initiate needed steps to ensure the sustainability of the coalition through the identification of funding sources for continued operation.

Review the goals mentioned in the text. List three to seven goals for your coalition in the first two years.

_____

_____

_____

_____

_____

_____

_____

_____

_____

_____

_____

IMPLEMENTING OBJECTIVES—ACTION ITEMS

After establishing coalition goals, the next step involves developing implementing objectives for each goal. These would include short-term targets for each goal that are measurable, realistic, and feasible and cover a period of one to two years. Specific steps are added in the form of action items, whereby specific tasks for achieving the objectives are identified along with assigning responsibility, accountability, and time frames. What follows are some example implementing objectives and action items for a healthcare emergency response coalition.

Goal: Ensure timely and effective communication between HERC members, the fiscal agent, member CEOs, elected officials, and the public.

Implementing Objectives: Design a communication plan to keep HERC members and other stakeholders updated on the activities of HERC.

Action Item 1: Develop an Internet-based calendar to notify members of upcoming meetings and events.

- Secure the appropriate web page and design the calendar.
- Update calendar with scheduled meetings and events.
- Notify members of the calendar location and any needed login IDs and passwords.

Due Date: January 30

Responsible Party: Coalition secretary

Action Item 2: Create a community report to distribute to the fiscal agent, member CEOs, elected officials, and the public.

- Gather content from coalition members.
- Secure outside graphic designer for layout (if needed).
- Secure outside printer (if needed).
- Distribute to appropriate stakeholders.
- Make electronic copy available in PDF format on website or through e-mail.

Due Date: August 1

Responsible Party: Communications committee chair

Review the goal, implementing objective, and action items in the text and develop implementing objectives and action items for each of your coalition goals. (A sample strategic plan and action plan are provided in Appendix D.)

_____

_____

_____

_____

_____

_____

_____

_____

_____

_____

_____

_____

_____

The above elements for development of a coalition's strategic plan are basic starting points. As the coalition progresses, members will find additional plan elements are needed. The key is to start with activities that are achievable and build confidence and pride among the members. Considerable time and effort should be devoted to the development of the strategic plan, with 100 percent buy-in by all coalition stakeholders.

DEVELOPING STANDARDIZED EMERGENCY OPERATING RESPONSE PROCEDURES

Homeland Security Presidential Directive (HSPD) 5 was released in 2003 to advance the capability of all agencies to be prepared for emergencies and disasters, and to collaborate and support each other more effectively through the continuum of mission areas.[1] The National Incident Management System (NIMS) implemented as part of HSPD-5 includes a template to guide agencies in working together and to coordinate federal, state, tribal, and local responder levels.[2] Hospitals and healthcare systems need to comply with NIMS if they receive federal preparedness and response grants, contracts, or cooperative agreement funds.[3] The national mission areas are:

- Prepare for response missions.
- Prevent, preempt, or deter acts of terrorism.
- Protect citizens, visitors, and critical infrastructure.
- Respond in an immediate, effective, and coordinated manner.
- Recover quickly and restore operations.

The Department of Homeland Security (DHS) issued guidelines for a National Response Framework (NRF) in 2008 that apply to all response agencies at every level, including hospitals and healthcare system facilities.[4] The goal for the NRF is to enable a unified national response that includes collaborating with other agencies, using common training, common language, and common preparation and responses to all-hazard types of events. The national preparedness guidelines support the capabilities-based planning process to define critical tasks and activities needed to accomplish each of the mission areas.[5]

Hospitals use a hospital incident command system (HICS) at their individual facilities to manage internal incidents, external threats, or actual events. HICS includes planning with external authorities and response agencies, including other hospitals, to ensure an integrated response. Command and control including the use of HICS can be evaluated during exercises and events to ensure that there is appropriate communication, responses are effective, and resources are applied as needed.

One of the benefits of a hospital and healthcare coalition is that common protocols can be developed as an all-hazards approach with hazard-specific management guidelines. Having a common operational approach to chemical, biological, radiological, nuclear, and explosive (CBRNE) threats will increase the consistency in the way hospitals prepare; prevent intentional or unintentional incidents; protect their facilities, staff, patients, and visitors; respond quickly and effectively; and recover quickly to maintain or regain the continuity of their operations.

For example, it is important that hospitals be aware of who is to be notified about reportable events and how the communication should occur to follow chains of established incident command pathways. Ensuring that the protocols can be implemented around the clock is critical, as disasters do not follow a daytime schedule.

Common protocols that coalitions can choose to develop include but are not limited to the following:

- Command and control
- Critical incident stress management
- Decontamination
- Donning and doffing
- Forensic evidence preservation and collection
- Management of contaminated materials
- Notification and communications
- Pharmaceutical cache management
- Reportable events hospital communication plan

A policy and procedures subcommittee that consists of multiple members of the HERC can be tasked with annual review of existing protocols and receive recommendations for new ones. The protocols are reviewed by local emergency management, public health, and key emergency response agencies so there is an understanding as to how incidents will be managed at coalition facilities.

The use of common communication systems and development of common protocols allows for sharing information with key response partners as to the capacity and capability of each coalition member. This may include a resource inventory of communication devices, personal protective equipment, specific disaster-related pharmaceuticals or equipment, bed census and surge space, location and staffing plans for alternate medical treatment sites, and others. Hospital coalitions are now using shared event management software that supports storage of protocols, inventories, and resource contact information to allow for internal HICS use and for sharing information with external partners as requested.

Major disasters can result in a need for evacuation of hospitals and healthcare systems or a local medical surge of patients. As part of a federal initiative entitled HAvBED (National Hospital Available Beds for Emergencies and Disasters), states are asked to request their hospitals and other healthcare systems to report on availability of specific types of beds such as adult intensive care unit beds, medical-surgical, psychiatric, pediatric, burn beds, and other types.[6] Other questions can be asked, such as the status of the facility in terms of demand and stress, equipment and supply availability, surge levels, or staffing needs, depending on the type of threat. States can facilitate entry of this information into a Web-based program that can be also viewed by local emergency authorities to anticipate resource needs, including transportation assets for emergency evacuation, cache supplies, or other resources.

Why would common protocols be helpful in a disaster response? Which protocols would best support a response in your area? List at least three.

_____

_____

_____

_____

_____

_____

_____

_____

_____

_____

_____

_____

_____

_____

_____

NOTES

1. www.dhs.gov/xabout/laws/gc_1214592333605.shtm (accessed October 7, 2009).

2. www.fema.gov/emergency/nims/index.shtm (accessed October 7, 2009).

3. NIMS: www.fema.gov/pdf/emergency/nims/hospital_faq.pdf (accessed October 7, 2009).

4. National Response Framework Resource Center: www.fema.gov/NRF (accessed October 5, 2009).

5. DHS National Preparedness Guidelines: www.dhs.gov/xlibrary/assets/National_Preparedness_Guidelines.pdf (accessed October 7, 2009).

6. HAvBED: www.innovations.ahrq.gov/content.aspx?id=753 (accessed October 7, 2009).

6

Sustainability: Keeping Your Coalition Going

Even though there is immediate value that a new healthcare emergency coalition will bring to its members and the community it serves, long-term sustainability should be a major consideration from the inception of the coalition. How much funding will be required in the first-year start-up? How will the coalition be supported in subsequent years? The answers will vary from community to community depending on the scope of the coalition's mission and its long-term strategic plan.

This chapter addresses financial sustainability methods to ensure long-term coalition viability. As noted earlier, the Healthcare Emergency Response Coalition (HERC) of Palm Beach County, Florida, was able to secure private foundation funding and in-kind donations from participating organizations at its inception. Initial money in 2001 was used to acquire hospital decontamination equipment, common communication systems, and for an external facilitator to assist with the development of a strategic plan, bylaws, and clinical protocols. By 2009 the Palm Beach County coalition's financial support came from the following five diverse funding sources:

- Local private foundation support
- Membership dues
- In-kind administrative support from member organizations
- Vendor sponsorship of monthly and annual meetings
- Sales of consulting services and other work products

Other coalitions have found other funding alternatives. The Miami-Dade County (Florida) Hospital Preparedness Consortium (www.mdchospitals.org/) receives grant support from the Miami-Dade County Health Department. The King County Healthcare Coalition in Seattle acquires substantial multiyear sustainability funding from the U.S. Department of Health and Human Services/Office of the Assistant Secretary of Preparedness and Response. These are just three examples of different revenue streams used in acquiring coalition support. The remainder of this chapter will explore a number of other funding options for long-term sustainability.

PHILANTHROPIC FUNDING

Foundations and other philanthropic organizations can provide seed money for initial start-up activities. Key steps for seeking this type of funding include:

- Identify and present information to a community-minded foundation, indicating how the coalition's activities will meet the funding entity's core mission.
- Delineate the multiple benefits the project will yield for both the community and the foundation.
- Provide a detailed evaluative methodology to measure success.
- Always publicize successful coalition efforts, which will demonstrate the stewardship of the funding foundation in the community.

The formation of a public affairs and sustainability committee or task force is extremely valuable in identifying not only philanthropic funding but also other types of funding sources.

FEDERAL GOVERNMENT FUNDING

Federal government funding may be secured from the U.S. Department of Homeland Security, the U.S. Department of Justice, and Urban Area Security Initiatives, as well as the Centers for Disease Control and Prevention and the U.S. Department of Health and Human Services. Remember, having multiple organizations partnering in a collaborative grant application is very attractive to all funders and gives the coalition significant advantages over a single organization applying for support.

LOCAL AND STATE GOVERNMENT FUNDING

While often not on the list of potential funding sources, local businesses and governments can and do provide resources for disaster preparedness projects. Again, it is best to approach these entities as a multiorganizational member coalition to maximize the chances of receiving funds. Examples of potential local governmental grant resources are:

- Municipalities
- County government (emergency management divisions)
- Healthcare districts
- County or state departments of health

MEMBERSHIP FEES

Another source of funding is by requiring annual membership dues. The initial amount may be minimal, but it would provide funds that the coalition can depend on during the start-up phase and subsequent years. To be viable, the benefits of membership must be worthwhile and must be seen as value added for the leadership team of the member organizations. In Palm Beach County the initial membership dues were $200 annually, which have increased annually to $500 per member as of 2009.

IN-KIND SERVICES

In-kind services can be of substantial assistance to a coalition. Member organizations may be able to donate personal protective equipment, provide decontamination training services, or offer administrative staffing support at little or no cost to the coalition. In Palm Beach County, support from county fire rescue services was invaluable to HERC in meeting the members' training needs. Also, during the early years, the Health Care District of Palm Beach County provided in-kind administrative support, which included distribution of minutes, archiving HERC documents, printing, and coordinating meeting schedules.

OTHER FUNDRAISING METHODS

As noted earlier, vendor sponsorship of monthly and annual meetings can raise considerable funds to support the coalition. The coalition member organizations represent millions of dollars in potential sales for a healthcare or emergency/disaster vendor. Do not underestimate this source of revenue to fund administrative costs of the coalition. In addition to vendor sponsorship, there may be opportunities for sales of consulting services or work products the coalition has generated. That is the case with HERC. The revenues generated from the sale of this book will be donated by the authors to the Healthcare Emergency Response Coalition of Palm Beach County, Florida, to ensure its sustainability.

EXCELLENT ACCOUNTING PROCEDURES

A component of financial sustainability is to ensure excellent accounting practices are in place. Not only is the coalition accountable to the membership, but as the coalition grows and acquires federal or other grants, considerable grant reporting will be required. Cooperative buying has proven very helpful to HERC by taking advantage of the coalition's volume purchasing power. In Palm Beach County, standardized purchases resulted in cost savings of 35 percent or more.

Although a number of potential coalition funding options have been discussed in this chapter, it is important to remember that the start-up of a coalition does not necessarily require a large amount of capital. The most important requirement for success is the time and effort the coalition member organizations' staff donate to the process. The commitment of the member organizations' staff time is the only essential requirement to begin the collaboration process.

Briefly address the following issues:

- How much financial support will your coalition need in the first year? Develop an initial working budget for the first year with detailed expenses listed.

- What legal entity will serve as the fiscal agent for your coalition?

- Will the coalition need to be an independent 501(c)(3) organization?

- List at least five potential revenue sources for your coalition. Be specific; if the resource is a foundation, what is the name of the foundation?

List at least five types of in-kind services that could be donated to your coalition (for example, meeting location). What specific entities, organizations, or members could provide these in-kind services?

_____

_____

_____

_____

_____

_____

_____

_____

_____

_____

_____

_____

_____

7

Top Ten Tips for Successful Coalition Building

This book has presented the organizational framework of the coalition as a proven model for healthcare organizations to partner together to address the many challenges a community faces. This chapter contains a summary in the format of a "Top Ten" list of tips for successful coalition building for emergency preparedness.

1. PARTNERING TO LEVERAGE RESOURCES

The coalition structure allows hospitals, physicians, nursing homes, dialysis providers, home health agencies, and other healthcare providers to partner together and work across organizational lines to prepare for and address critical challenges facing a community. Doing so provides the opportunity to leverage resources by combining the expertise of multiorganization staff and the ability to share the financial burden of large community-wide projects, which ultimately provides individual organizations with a return on their "investment" that far outweighs their individual contribution. The healthcare coalition structure demonstrates a willingness by the healthcare community to come to the table as a partner to address the many challenges a community might face. As a result, coalitions enable the healthcare community to partner with the emergency preparedness community to optimally prepare for all challenges.

2. COMMUNITY SUPPORT

Foster community support early. When healthcare organizations form a coalition, it enables them to generate additional support from the community. Local governments and emergency response professionals are often motivated to leverage their resources to help further expand hospital, physician, and provider capabilities to respond to a disaster event. In addition, local and state politicians are better positioned to bring resources to a community when they can demonstrate a true collaborative approach through a coalition. Community support at the beginning can help identify a financial champion, like a local or national foundation, that can help fund the activities of the coalition. Foundations generally find that grants to large groups partnering together can maximize their dollars, as opposed to single entities working on more narrow projects.

3. COMMUNITY-WIDE HAZARD VULNERABILITY ASSESSMENT

Community or joint hazard vulnerability assessments are a great early activity for a new coalition. Ranking a list of hazards, the probability of their occurrence, the impact they might have, and the preparedness level and capability of the community to manage such threats can help guide a new coalition on the types of training and exercises that should be prioritized. The joint hazard vulnerability assessment should be conducted with local emergency management and response partners.

4. COMMON COMMUNICATIONS SYSTEMS

Communication is one of the most important factors that dictate the success of a coalition and the response partners during a disaster event. Coalitions should select and use common systems for threat notification, activations, and routine sharing of information about meetings, training, and resources. Generating a common contact list, using event management software, reporting bed availability, and many other communication tools are all important to keeping a coalition functioning.

5. JOINT TRAINING AND EXERCISES

Coalitions should always try to train and exercise together. Shared training sessions should include core competencies such as disaster awareness, operations level training, decontamination, use of communication systems, community mass care management, critical infrastructure assessment and protection, risk communications, disaster behavioral health training, continuity of operations planning (COOP), and a range of others that are all-hazards and hazard-specific. At least one joint exercise should be planned by coalition members and executed each year. The coalition can generate a list of objectives that are hospital- or healthcare group–specific, in addition to each hospital adding objectives that they specifically need to test. Typically, each coalition will identify an exercise committee that actively participates in the joint planning sessions with emergency management and response partners.

6. ENLISTING SUPPORT OF CEOs

One of the most important groups to garner support from is the CEOs and directors from the coalition's members. The long-term viability and success of the coalition can hinge on the level of engagement and interest from the CEOs. Staff time and financial resources are a large commitment from any organization. Including the CEOs in the early planning stages and taking the time and effort to keep them updated and involved in the coalition's activities is one of the surest ways to enlist their support.

7. DESIGNATING THE ORGANIZATION'S REPRESENTATIVES

The optimal professional mix or makeup of the coalition is very important. For example, the coalition should target the types of professions and disciplines that will bring the needed expertise to the coalition. For hospital members, the infection control practitioner, emergency preparedness coordinator, and safety officer all have skill sets that would bring value to the coalition. Within the mix, it is also valuable for some hospitals to include representatives from administration, like a chief operating officer.

8. CHOOSING A FISCAL AGENT

The choice of a fiscal agent is another important decision that should be made with great care. A fiscal agent is needed for the coalition because state, federal, and foundation grantors require a legal entity to receive funding. A fiscal agent will enable a coalition to apply for funding, fully benefit from group purchasing, and reconcile financial matters.

9. TRANSFORMATIONAL LEADERSHIP

The chairperson for the coalition should possess transformational leadership qualities. This individual must be able to bring together many diverse functions, including strategic planning, assessment and reassessment of goals, developing agendas for committee and membership meetings, facilitating discussions, and serving as the voice of the coalition to represent the healthcare mission within emergency response. The type of leader who would be a good fit for a healthcare emergency response coalition is someone who, among many talents, is:

- A member of the healthcare community, preferably from an accredited hospital
- Familiar with hospital and healthcare regulatory standards, including state and federal guidance
- Experienced in being actively involved with hospital and community disaster planning and response, preferably with experience serving in a role within his or her own hospital incident command system structure
- Has good communication skills

10. SUSTAINABILITY

One of the primary challenges that will face a coalition is how to sustain the good work and operations of the group. Planning for sustainability from the beginning is very important. Funding for administration and operations is often difficult to come by and should be incorporated into the early plans of the coalition. In addition to funding, succession planning for chairpersons, committee members, and new designated representatives from member organizations should be a priority. Having these plans in place will help ensure the smooth transition from one leader to the next, one hospital representative to the next, and so forth.

List of Appendixes

For more resources and samples, please visit the Palm Beach County Medical Society Healthcare Emergency Response Coalition website at www.pbcms.org/herc.

Appendix A

Glossary of NIMS Terms

For the purposes of the National Incident Management System (NIMS), the following terms and definitions apply. (Source: dma.mt.gov/des/Library/NIMS/GLOSSARY.pdf.)

Agency: A division of government with a specific function offering a particular kind of assistance. In ICS, agencies are defined either as jurisdictional (having statutory responsibility for incident management) or as assisting or cooperating (providing resources or other assistance).

Agency Representative: A person assigned by a primary, assisting, or cooperating state, local, or tribal government agency or private entity that has been delegated authority to make decisions affecting that agency's or organization's participation in incident management activities following appropriate consultation with the leadership of that agency.

Area Command (Unified Area Command): An organization established (1) to oversee the management of multiple incidents that are each being handled by an ICS organization or (2) to oversee the management of large or multiple incidents to which several Incident Management Teams have been assigned. Area Command has the responsibility to set overall strategy and priorities, allocate critical resources according to priorities, ensure that incidents are properly managed, and ensure that objectives are met and strategies followed. Area Command becomes Unified Area Command when incidents are multijurisdictional. Area Command may be established at an emergency operations center facility or at some location other than an incident command post.

Assessment: The evaluation and interpretation of measurements and other information to provide a basis for decision-making.

Assignments: Tasks given to resources to perform within a given operational period that are based on operational objectives defined in the IAP.

Assistant: Title for subordinates of principal Command Staff positions. The title indicates a level of technical capability, qualifications, and responsibility subordinate to the primary positions. Assistants may also be assigned to unit leaders.

Assisting Agency: An agency or organization providing personnel, services, or other resources to the agency with direct responsibility for incident management.

Available Resources: Resources assigned to an incident, checked in, and available for a mission assignment, normally located in a Staging Area.

Branch: The organizational level having functional or geographical responsibility for major aspects of incident operations. A branch is organizationally situated between the section and the division or group in the Operations Section, and between the section and units in the Logistics Section. Branches are identified by the use of Roman numerals or by functional area.

Chain of Command: A series of command, control, executive, or management positions in hierarchical order of authority.

Check-In: The process through which resources first report to an incident. Check-in locations include the incident command post, Resources Unit, incident base, camps, staging areas, or directly on the site.

Chief: The ICS title for individuals responsible for management of functional sections: Operations, Planning, Logistics, Finance/Administration, and Intelligence (if established as a separate section).

Command: The act of directing, ordering, or controlling by virtue of explicit statutory, regulatory, or delegated authority.

Command Staff: In an incident management organization, the Command Staff consists of the Incident Command and the special staff positions of Public Information Officer, Safety Officer, Liaison Officer, and other positions as required, who report directly to the Incident Commander. They may have an assistant or assistants, as needed.

Common Operating Picture: A broad view of the overall situation as reflected by situation reports, aerial photography, and other information or intelligence.

Communications Unit: An organizational unit in the Logistics Section responsible for providing communication services at an incident or an Emergency Operations Center (EOC). A Communications Unit may also be a facility (e.g., a trailer or mobile van) used to support an Incident Communications Center.

Cooperating Agency: An agency supplying assistance other than direct operational or support functions or resources to the incident management effort.

Coordinate: To advance systematically an analysis and exchange of information among principals who have or may have a need to know certain information to carry out specific incident management responsibilities.

Deputy: A fully qualified individual who, in the absence of a superior, can be delegated the authority to manage a functional operation or perform a specific task. In some cases, a deputy can act as relief for a superior and, therefore, must be fully qualified in the position. Deputies can be assigned to the Incident Commander, General Staff, and Branch Directors.

Dispatch: The ordered movement of a resource or resources to an assigned operational mission or an administrative move from one location to another.

Division: The partition of an incident into geographical areas of operation. Divisions are established when the number of resources exceeds the manageable span of control of the Operations Chief. A division is located within the ICS organization between the branch and resources in the Operations Section.

Emergency: Absent a Presidentially declared emergency, any incident(s), human-caused or natural, that requires responsive action to protect life or property. Under the Robert T. Stafford Disaster Relief and Emergency Assistance Act, an emergency means any occasion or instance for which, in the determination of the President, Federal assistance is needed to supplement State and local efforts and capabilities to save lives and to protect property and public health and safety, or to lessen or avert the threat of a catastrophe in any part of the United States.

Emergency Operations Centers (EOCs): The physical location at which the coordination of information and resources to support domestic incident management activities normally takes place. An EOC may be a temporary facility or may be located in a more central or permanently established facility, perhaps at a higher level of organization within a jurisdiction. EOCs may be organized by major functional disciplines (e.g., fire, law enforcement, and medical services), by jurisdiction (e.g., Federal, State, regional, county, city, tribal), or some combination thereof.

Emergency Operations Plan: The "steady-state" plan maintained by various jurisdictional levels for responding to a wide variety of potential hazards.

Emergency Public Information: Information that is disseminated primarily in anticipation of an emergency or during an emergency. In addition to providing situational information to the public, it also frequently provides directive actions required to be taken by the general public.

Emergency Response Provider: Includes state, local, and tribal emergency public safety, law enforcement, emergency response, emergency medical (including hospital emergency facilities), and related personnel, agencies, and authorities. See Section 2 (6), Homeland Security Act of 2002, Pub. L. 107-296, 116 Stat. 2135 (2002). Also known as *Emergency Responder*.

Evacuation: Organized, phased, and supervised withdrawal, dispersal, or removal of civilians from dangerous or potentially dangerous areas, and their reception and care in safe areas.

Event: A planned, nonemergency activity. ICS can be used as the management system for a wide range of events, e.g., parades, concerts, or sporting events.

Federal: Of or pertaining to the Federal Government of the United States of America.

Function: Function refers to the five major activities in ICS: Command, Operations, Planning, Logistics, and Finance/Administration. The term function is also used when describing the activity involved, e.g., the planning function. A sixth function, Intelligence, may be established, if required, to meet incident management needs.

General Staff: A group of incident management personnel organized according to function and reporting to the Incident Commander. The General Staff normally consists of the Operations Section Chief, Planning Section Chief, Logistics Section Chief, and Finance/Administration Section Chief.

Group: Established to divide the incident management structure into functional areas of operation. Groups are composed of resources assembled to perform a special function not necessarily within a single geographic division. Groups, when activated, are located between branches and resources in the Operations Section. (See *Division*.)

Hazard: Something that is potentially dangerous or harmful, often the root cause of an unwanted outcome.

Incident: An occurrence or event, natural or human-caused, that requires an emergency response to protect life or property. Incidents can, for example, include major disasters, emergencies, terrorist attacks, terrorist threats, wildland and urban fires, floods, hazardous materials spills, nuclear accidents, aircraft accidents, earthquakes, hurricanes, tornadoes, tropical storms, war-related disasters, public health and medical emergencies, and other occurrences requiring an emergency response.

Incident Action Plan: An oral or written plan containing general objectives reflecting the overall strategy for managing an incident. It may include the identification of operational resources and assignments. It may also include attachments that provide direction and important information for management of the incident during one or more operational periods.

Incident Command Post (ICP): The field location at which the primary tactical-level, on-scene incident command functions are performed. The ICP may be collocated with the incident base or other incident facilities and is normally identified by a green rotating or flashing light.

Incident Command System (ICS): A standardized on-scene emergency management construct specifically designed to provide for the adoption of an integrated organizational structure that reflects the complexity and demands of single or multiple incidents, without being hindered by jurisdictional boundaries. ICS is the combination of facilities, equipment, personnel, procedures, and communications operating within a common organizational structure, designed to aid in the management of resources during incidents. It is used for all kinds of emergencies and is applicable to small as well as large and complex incidents. ICS is used by various jurisdictions and functional agencies, both public and private, to organize field-level incident management operations.

Incident Commander (IC): The individual responsible for all incident activities, including the development of strategies and tactics and the ordering and the release of resources. The IC has overall authority and responsibility for conducting incident operations and is responsible for the management of all incident operations at the incident site.

Incident Management Team (IMT): The IC and appropriate Command and General Staff personnel assigned to an incident.

Incident Objectives: Statements of guidance and direction necessary for selecting appropriate strategy(s) and the tactical direction of resources. Incident objectives are based on realistic expectations of what can be accomplished when all allocated resources have been effectively deployed. Incident objectives must be achievable and measurable, yet flexible enough to allow strategic and tactical alternatives.

Initial Action: The actions taken by those responders first to arrive at an incident site.

Initial Response: Resources initially committed to an incident.

Intelligence Officer: The intelligence officer is responsible for managing internal information, intelligence, and operational security requirements supporting incident management activities. These may include information security and operational security activities, as well as the complex task of ensuring that sensitive information of all types (e.g., classified information, law enforcement sensitive information, proprietary information, or export-controlled information) is handled in a way that not only safeguards the information, but also ensures that it gets to those who need access to it to perform their missions effectively and safely.

Joint Information Center (JIC): A facility established to coordinate all incident-related public information activities. It is the central point of contact for all news media at the scene of the incident. Public information officials from all participating agencies should collocate at the JIC.

Joint Information System (JIS): Integrates incident information and public affairs into a cohesive organization designed to provide consistent, coordinated, timely information during crisis or incident operations. The mission of the JIS is to provide a structure and system for developing and delivering coordinated interagency messages; developing, recommending, and executing public information plans and strategies on behalf of the IC; advising the IC concerning public affairs issues that could affect a response effort; and controlling rumors and inaccurate information that could undermine public confidence in the emergency response effort.

Jurisdiction: A range or sphere of authority. Public agencies have jurisdiction at an incident related to their legal responsibilities and authority. Jurisdictional authority at an incident can be political or geographical (e.g., city, county, tribal, State, or Federal boundary lines) or functional (e.g., law enforcement, public health).

Liaison: A form of communication for establishing and maintaining mutual understanding and cooperation.

Liaison Officer: A member of the Command Staff responsible for coordinating with representatives from cooperating and assisting agencies.

Local Government: A county, municipality, city, town, township, local public authority, school district, special district, intrastate district, council of governments (regardless of whether the council of governments is incorporated as a nonprofit corporation under State law), regional or interstate government entity, or agency or instrumentality of a local government; an Indian tribe or authorized tribal organization, or in Alaska a Native village or Alaska Regional Native Corporation; a rural community, unincorporated town or village, or other public entity. See Section 2 (10), Homeland Security Act of 2002, Pub. L. 107-296, 116 Stat. 2135 (2002).

Logistics: Providing resources and other services to support incident management.

Logistics Section: The section responsible for providing facilities, services, and material support for the incident.

Major Disaster: As defined under the Robert T. Stafford Disaster Relief and Emergency Assistance Act (42 U.S.C. 5122), a major disaster is any natural catastrophe (including any hurricane, tornado, storm, high water, wind-driven water, tidal wave, tsunami, earthquake, volcanic eruption, landslide, mudslide, snowstorm, or drought), or, regardless of cause, any fire, flood, or explosion, in any part of the United States, which in the determination of the President causes damage of sufficient severity and magnitude to warrant major disaster assistance under this Act to supplement the efforts and available resources of States, tribes, local governments, and disaster relief organizations in alleviating the damage, loss, hardship, or suffering caused thereby.

Management by Objective: A management approach that involves a four-step process for achieving the incident goal. The Management by Objectives approach includes the following: establishing overarching objectives; developing and issuing assignments, plans, procedures, and protocols; establishing specific, measurable objectives for various incident management functional activities and directing efforts to fulfill them, in support of defined strategic objectives; and documenting results to measure performance and facilitate corrective action.

Mitigation: The activities designed to reduce or eliminate risks to persons or property or to lessen the actual or potential effects or consequences of an incident. Mitigation measures may be implemented prior to, during, or after an incident. Mitigation measures are often informed by lessons learned from prior incidents. Mitigation involves ongoing actions to reduce exposure to, probability of, or potential loss from hazards. Measures may include zoning and building codes, floodplain buyouts, and analysis of hazard-related data to determine where it is safe to build or locate temporary facilities. Mitigation can include efforts to educate governments, businesses, and the public on measures they can take to reduce loss and injury.

Mobilization: The process and procedures used by all organizations—state, local, and tribal—for activating, assembling, and transporting all resources that have been requested to respond to or support an incident.

Multiagency Coordination Entity: A multiagency coordination entity functions within a broader multiagency coordination system. It may establish the priorities among incidents and associated resource allocations, deconflict agency policies, and provide strategic guidance and direction to support incident management activities.

Multiagency Coordination Systems: Multiagency coordination systems provide the architecture to support coordination for incident prioritization, critical resource allocation, communications systems integration, and information coordination. The components of multiagency coordination systems include facilities, equipment, emergency operation centers (EOCs), specific multiagency coordination entities, personnel, procedures, and communications. These systems assist agencies and organizations to fully integrate the subsystems of the NIMS.

Multijurisdictional Incident: An incident requiring action from multiple agencies that each have jurisdiction to manage certain aspects of an incident. In ICS, these incidents will be managed under Unified Command.

Mutual-Aid Agreement: Written agreement between agencies and/or jurisdictions that they will assist one another on request, by furnishing personnel, equipment, and/or expertise in a specified manner.

National: Of a nationwide character, including the state, local, and tribal aspects of governance and policy.

National Disaster Medical System (NDMS): A cooperative, asset-sharing partnership between the Department of Health and Human Services, the Department of Veterans Affairs, the Department of Homeland Security, and the Department of Defense. NDMS provides resources for meeting the continuity of care and mental health services requirements of the Emergency Support Function 8 in the Federal Response Plan.

National Incident Management System (NIMS): A system mandated by Homeland Security Presidential Directive 5 (HSPD-5) that provides a consistent nationwide approach for state, local, and tribal governments; the private-sector, and nongovernmental organizations to work effectively and efficiently together to prepare for, respond to, and recover from domestic incidents, regardless of cause, size, or complexity. To provide for interoperability and compatibility among state, local, and tribal capabilities, the NIMS includes a core set of concepts, principles, and terminology. HSPD-5 identifies these as the ICS; multiagency coordination systems; training; identification and management of resources (including systems for classifying types of resources); qualification and certification; and the collection, tracking, and reporting of incident information and incident resources.

National Response Plan: A plan mandated by HSPD-5 that integrates Federal domestic prevention, preparedness, response, and recovery plans into one all-discipline, all-hazards plan.

Nongovernmental Organization: An entity with an association that is based on interests of its members, individuals, or institutions and that is not created by a government, but may work cooperatively with government. Such organizations serve a public purpose, not a private benefit. Examples of NGOs include faith-based charity organizations and the American Red Cross.

Operational Period: The time scheduled for executing a given set of operation actions, as specified in the Incident Action Plan. Operational periods can be of various lengths, although usually not over 24 hours.

Operations Section: The section responsible for all tactical incident operations. In ICS, it normally includes subordinate branches, divisions, and/or groups.

Personnel Accountability: The ability to account for the location and welfare of incident personnel. It is accomplished when supervisors ensure that ICS principles and processes are functional and that personnel are working within established incident management guidelines.

Planning Meeting: A meeting held as needed prior to and throughout the duration of an incident to select specific strategies and tactics for incident control operations and for service and support planning. For larger incidents, the planning meeting is a major element in the development of the Incident Action Plan (IAP).

Planning Section: Responsible for the collection, evaluation, and dissemination of operational information related to the incident, and for the preparation and documentation of the IAP. This section also maintains information on the current and forecasted situation and on the status of resources assigned to the incident.

Preparedness: The range of deliberate, critical tasks and activities necessary to build, sustain, and improve the operational capability to prevent, protect against, respond to, and recover from domestic incidents. Preparedness is a continuous process. Preparedness involves efforts at all levels of government and between government and private-sector and nongovernmental organizations to identify threats, determine vulnerabilities, and identify required resources. Within the NIMS, preparedness is operationally focused on establishing guidelines, protocols, and standards for planning, training and exercises, personnel qualification and certification, equipment certification, and publication management.

Preparedness Organizations: The groups and forums that provide interagency coordination for domestic incident management activities in a nonemergency context. Preparedness organizations can include all agencies with a role in incident management, for prevention, preparedness, response, or recovery activities. They represent a wide variety of committees, planning groups, and other organizations that meet and coordinate to ensure the proper level of planning, training, equipping, and other preparedness requirements within a jurisdiction or area.

Prevention: Actions to avoid an incident or to intervene to stop an incident from occurring. Prevention involves actions to protect lives and property. It involves applying intelligence and other information to a range of activities that may include such countermeasures as deterrence operations; heightened inspections; improved surveillance and security operations; investigations to determine the full nature and source of the threat; public health and agricultural surveillance and testing processes; immunizations, isolation, or quarantine; and, as appropriate, specific law enforcement operations aimed at deterring, preempting, interdicting, or disrupting illegal activity and apprehending potential perpetrators and bringing them to justice.

Private Sector: Organizations and entities that are not part of any governmental structure. It includes for-profit and not-for-profit organizations, formal and informal structures, commerce and industry, and private voluntary organizations (PVO).

Processes: Systems of operations that incorporate standardized procedures, methodologies, and functions necessary to provide resources effectively and efficiently. These include resource typing, resource ordering and tracking, and coordination.

Public Information Officer: A member of the Command Staff responsible for interfacing with the public and media or with other agencies with incident-related information requirements.

Publications Management: The publications management subsystem includes materials development, publication control, publication supply, and distribution. The development and distribution of NIMS materials is managed through this subsystem. Consistent documentation is critical to success, because it ensures that all responders are familiar with the documentation used in a particular incident regardless of the location or the responding agencies involved.

Qualification and Certification: This subsystem provides recommended qualification and certification standards for emergency responder and incident management personnel. It also allows the development of minimum standards for resources expected to have an interstate application. Standards typically include training, currency, experience, and physical and medical fitness.

Reception Area: This refers to a location separate from staging areas, where resources report in for processing and out-processing. Reception Areas provide accountability, security, situational awareness briefings, safety awareness, distribution of IAPs, supplies and equipment, feeding, and bed down.

Recovery: The development, coordination, and execution of service- and site-restoration plans; the reconstitution of government operations and services; individual, private-sector, nongovernmental, and public-assistance programs to provide housing and to promote restoration; long-term care and treatment of affected persons; additional measures for social, political, environmental, and economic restoration; evaluation of the incident to identify lessons learned; postincident reporting; and development of initiatives to mitigate the effects of future incidents.

Recovery Plan: A plan developed by a State, local, or tribal jurisdiction with assistance from responding Federal agencies to restore the affected area.

Resources: Personnel and major items of equipment, supplies, and facilities available or potentially available for assignment to incident operations and for which status is maintained. Resources are described by kind and type and may be used in operational support or supervisory capacities at an incident or at an EOC.

Resource Management: Efficient incident management requires a system for identifying available resources at all jurisdictional levels to enable timely and unimpeded access to resources needed to prepare for, respond to, or recover from an incident. Resource management under the NIMS includes mutual-aid agreements; the use of special state, local, and tribal teams; and resource mobilization protocols.

Resources Unit: Functional unit within the Planning Section responsible for recording the status of resources committed to the incident. This unit also evaluates resources currently committed to the incident, the effects additional responding resources will have on the incident, and anticipated resource needs.

Response: Activities that address the short-term, direct effects of an incident. Response includes immediate actions to save lives, protect property, and meet basic human needs. Response also includes the execution of emergency operations plans and of mitigation activities designed to limit the loss of life, personal injury, property damage, and other unfavorable outcomes. As indicated by the situation, response activities include applying intelligence and other information to lessen the effects or consequences of an incident; increased security operations; continuing investigations into nature and source of the threat; ongoing public health and agricultural surveillance and testing processes; immunizations, isolation, or quarantine; and specific law enforcement operations aimed at preempting, interdicting, or disrupting illegal activity, and apprehending actual perpetrators and bringing them to justice.

Safety Officer: A member of the Command Staff responsible for monitoring and assessing safety hazards or unsafe situations and for developing measures for ensuring personnel safety.

Section: The organizational level having responsibility for a major functional area of incident management, e.g., Operations, Planning, Logistics, Finance/Administration, and Intelligence (if established). The section is organizationally situated between the branch and the Incident Command.

Span of Control: The number of individuals a supervisor is responsible for, usually expressed as the ratio of supervisors to individuals. (Under the NIMS, an appropriate span of control is between 1:3 and 1:7.)

Staging Area: Location established where resources can be placed while awaiting a tactical assignment. The Operations Section manages Staging Areas.

State: When capitalized, refers to any State of the United States, the District of Columbia, the Commonwealth of Puerto Rico, the Virgin Islands, Guam, American Samoa, the Commonwealth of the Northern Mariana Islands, and any possession of the United States. See Section 2 (14), Homeland Security Act of 2002, Pub. L. 107-296, 116 Stat. 2135 (2002).

Strategic: Strategic elements of incident management are characterized by continuous long-term, high-level planning by organizations headed by elected or other senior officials. These elements involve the adoption of long-range goals and objectives, the setting of priorities; the establishment of budgets and other fiscal decisions, policy development, and the application of measures of performance or effectiveness.

Strategy: The general direction selected to accomplish incident objectives set by the IC.

Strike Team: A set number of resources of the same kind and type that have an established minimum number of personnel.

Supporting Technologies: Any technology that may be used to support the NIMS is included in this subsystem. These technologies include orthophoto mapping, remote automatic weather stations, infrared technology, and communications, among various others.

Task Force: Any combination of resources assembled to support a specific mission or operational need. All resource elements within a Task Force must have common communications and a designated leader.

Technical Assistance: Support provided to State, local, and tribal jurisdictions when they have the resources but lack the complete knowledge and skills needed to perform a required activity (such as mobile-home park design and hazardous material assessments).

Terrorism: Under the Homeland Security Act of 2002, terrorism is defined as activity that involves an act dangerous to human life or potentially destructive of critical infrastructure or key resources and is a violation of the criminal laws of the United States or of any State or other subdivision of the United States in which it occurs and is intended to intimidate or coerce the civilian population or influence a government or affect the conduct of a government by mass destruction, assassination, or kidnapping. See Section 2 (15), Homeland Security Act of 2002, Pub. L. 107-296, 116 Stat. 2135 (2002).

Threat: An indication of possible violence, harm, or danger.

Tools: Those instruments and capabilities that allow for the professional performance of tasks, such as information systems, agreements, doctrine, capabilities, and legislative authorities.

Tribal: Any Indian tribe, band, nation, or other organized group or community, including any Alaskan Native Village as defined in or established pursuant to the Alaskan Native Claims Settlement Act (85 stat. 688) [43 U.S.C.A. and 1601 et seq.], that is recognized as eligible for the special programs and services provided by the United States to Indians because of their status as Indians.

Type: A classification of resources in the ICS that refers to capability. Type 1 is generally considered to be more capable than Types 2, 3, or 4, respectively, because of size; power; capacity; or, in the case of incident management teams, experience and qualifications.

Unified Area Command: A Unified Area Command is established when incidents under an Area Command are multijurisdictional. (See *Area Command.*)

Unified Command (UC): An application of ICS used when there is more than one agency with incident jurisdiction or when incidents cross political jurisdictions. Agencies work together through the designated members of the UC, often the senior person from agencies and/or disciplines participating in the UC, to establish a common set of objectives and strategies and a single IAP.

Unit: The organizational element having functional responsibility for a specific incident planning, logistics, or finance/administration activity.

Unity of Command: The concept by which each person within an organization reports to one and only one designated person. The purpose of unity of command is to ensure unity of effort under one responsible commander for every objective.

Volunteer: For purposes of the NIMS, a volunteer is any individual accepted to perform services by the lead agency, which has authority to accept volunteer services, when the individual performs services without promise, expectation, or receipt of compensation for services performed. See, e.g., 16 U.S.C. 742f(c) and 29 CFR 553.101.

Appendix B

Memorandum of Understanding (MOU) (Sample)

**Healthcare Emergency Response Coalition of Palm Beach County
Mutual Aid Memorandum of Understanding
Sample**

This Healthcare Emergency Response Coalition of Palm Beach County (HERC) Mutual Aid
Memorandum of Understanding ("MOU") is made effective this _____day of _____ 2004 by and
between the Healthcare Facilities listed below as signatories to this MOU.

I.   Introduction and Background

As one of the nation's premier recreation and international business locations, Palm Beach County is
susceptible to disasters, both natural and man-made, that could consequently exceed the resources of any
individual hospital. A disaster may require specialized medical resources (i.e., trauma surgery, pulmonary
care, resources required to treat hazmat injuries), and the required resources may exceed the capacity of
the Impacted Facility; or a disaster/incident may involve building damage, physical plant problems,
and/or utility failure resulting in the need for partial or complete hospital evacuation.

This document addresses the relationships between and among healthcare facilities and is intended to
augment, not replace, each facility's emergency management/disaster plan. The MOU also provides the
framework for healthcare facilities to coordinate as a single Healthcare Facility Mutual Aid System
(HFMAS) community in coordination with Palm Beach County Emergency Management (PBCEM),
Palm Beach County Health Department (PBCHD), and Palm Beach County EMS (municipal and private
sector) during planning and response. This document does not replace but rather supplements the rules
and procedures governing interaction with other organizations during a Disaster, e.g., law enforcement
agencies, the Florida Department of Emergency Management, Florida Department of Health, fire
departments, American Red Cross, etc.

II.   Purpose of Mutual Aid Memorandum of Understanding

This MOU is a voluntary agreement among the Healthcare Facility members of Palm Beach County for
the purpose of providing mutual aid at the time of a Disaster that requires the professional assistance of
one or more Healthcare Facility members. The purpose of this MOU is for participating Healthcare
Facilities to aid each other in their emergency management by authorizing the "HFMAS." HFMAS
addresses the loan of medical personnel, pharmaceuticals, supplies, and equipment, or assistance with
emergency Healthcare Facility evacuation, including accepting transferred patients.

III.   Definition of Terms

Command Post	An area established in a Healthcare Facility for use during an emergency that is a primary source of administrative authority by administrative personnel to make decisions relative to the emergency.
Communication Center	The location within a Healthcare Facility through which information is collected and reported to MedComm.

Disaster	A Disaster is defined as an overwhelming incident that exceeds the effective response capability of the Impacted Healthcare Facility or Facilities. An incident of this magnitude will almost always involve Palm Beach County Emergency Management (PBCEM) and the Palm Beach County Health Department (PBCHD) and may involve loan of medical and support personnel, pharmaceuticals, supplies, and equipment from another facility or the assistance with emergency evacuation of patients of the Impacted Healthcare Facility. The Disaster may result from an "external" or "internal" event for the Impacted Healthcare Facility. The definition of Disaster assumes that each Impacted Healthcare Facility's emergency management plan has been fully implemented.
Donor Facility	The Healthcare Facility that provides personnel, pharmaceuticals, supplies, and/or equipment to an Impacted Facility experiencing a disaster.
EOC ESF#8–Health and Medical	The Emergency Operations Center—the location established by each jurisdiction to centralize coordination of all aspects of a Disaster response. ESF#8–Health and Medical will be responsible for coordinating all health and medical and veterinarian related assistance. The Palm Beach County Health Department is the lead coordinating agency for ESF#8–Health and Medical.
HERC	The 15 hospitals who are parties to this MOU—along with representatives from public safety, public health, mental health, and emergency management—who meet to plan, train, and exercise together in order to best assure a coordinated, timely and effective response to a Disaster.
HFMAS	The Healthcare Facility Mutual Aid System, through which participating facilities will loan services and items, including personnel, pharmaceuticals, supplies, equipment, and/or such other assistance to an Impacted Facility.
HMACS	The Hospital Mutual Aid Communication System, the primary communication system (UHF (MedComm)-800 MHz radio, telephone, fax etc.) used by healthcare facilities to communicate with the EOC and each other during a Disaster.
HMARS	The Hospital Mutual Aid Radio System, a secondary radio communication system used by MedComm/HERC and ESF#8 through which communication can take place during an emergency with county hospitals.
Impacted Healthcare Facility	The Healthcare Facility where the Disaster occurred or the place where Disaster victims are being treated.
JIC	The Joint Information Center, the location established by the county, state, and/or federal government to coordinate the release of information to the press, media, and general public. Each Healthcare Facility agrees to participate in providing information to the JIC and help to convey a unified message developed for release to the public.

MedComm	A communication and information system that has 800 MHz capability and UHF network, which allows communication to take place between Healthcare Facilities and Emergency Responders to immediately make available Healthcare Facility resources at the time of a Disaster. MedComm is operational 24 hours a day and requires daily maintenance during a Disaster. MedComm does have limited decision-making and supervisory authority and principally collects and disseminates information and performs regular checks of the HMACS system. Florida State EMS Communications refers to MedComm as Medical Control Center (MCC), and it can be found in Appendix E of Volume 1 of the State Plan.
Participating Hospitals	Healthcare Facilities that have committed to HFMAS and are parties to this MOU.
Partner	The designated facility (or healthcare system) that an Impacted Healthcare Facility communicates with as such facility's "first call for help" during a Disaster. Partners may be developed through an optional Partnering arrangement.
Patient Receiving Facility	The Healthcare Facility that receives transferred patients from an Impacted Facility responding to a Disaster.
Patient Transferring Facility	An Impacted Healthcare Facility that evacuates patients to a Patient-Receiving Facility in response to a Disaster.
Recipient Facility	An Impacted Facility that has requested personnel or materials from another Healthcare Facility.

IV.   General Principles of Understanding

1.   <u>Participating Healthcare Facilities:</u> Each Healthcare Facility agrees to designate a primary and alternate representative to attend the HERC meetings and coordinate the mutual aid initiatives in accordance with the individual Healthcare Facility's emergency preparedness/management plans. Healthcare Facilities also agree to commit to participate in HFMAS exercises and maintain their communication links to MEDCOMM/ HMACS.

2.   <u>Partnering:</u> Each Healthcare Facility, in its sole discretion, may partner with another Healthcare Facility that shall be the "first call for help" during a Disaster. The Healthcare Facilities that agree to become Partners shall develop, prior to any Disaster, methods for coordinating communication between each other, responding to the media, and identifying the locations to enter their Partner Healthcare Facility's security perimeter.

Each Partnered Healthcare Facility should standardize a set of contacts to facilitate communications during a Disaster in conjunction with the HERC.

The procedural steps in the event of a disaster are as follows:

   a.   Impacted Healthcare Facility contacts MedComm and/or ESF-8 when activated and notifies the center of its needs, how they are being met, and any unmet needs.
   b.   At the request of the Impacted Healthcare Facility, MedComm and/or ESF-8 will contact other Healthcare Facilities to alert them of the situation and to begin an inventory for any possible or actual unmet needs.

c. The facilities shall determine the total number of patients the emergency department and Healthcare Facility can accept, and if possible, the total number of patients with major and minor injuries.

d. Impacted Healthcare Facility contacts Partner Healthcare Facility to determine availability of beds, equipment, supplies, and personnel. (Contacts secondary Partner Facility if primary Partner Facility is unable to meet needs.)

3. Implementation of MOU: During a Disaster, only the authorized administrator (or designee) or Command Center at each Healthcare Facility has the authority to request or offer assistance through HMACS. Communications between Healthcare Facilities for formally requesting and volunteering assistance shall be conducted among the senior administrators (or designees) or respective Command Centers.

4. Healthcare Facility: The Impacted Facility's Command Center is responsible for informing MedComm/ESF#8–Health and Medical of its situation and defining needs that cannot be accommodated by the Healthcare Facility itself or any existing Partner Facility. The senior administrator or designee is responsible for requesting personnel, pharmaceuticals, supplies, equipment, or authorizing the evacuation of patients. The senior administrator or designee will coordinate, both internally and with the Donor/Patient-Accepting Facility/ESF#8–Health and Medical (when activated), all of the logistics involved in implementing assistance under this MOU. Logistics include identifying the number and specific location where personnel, pharmaceuticals, supplies, equipment, or patients should be sent, how to enter the security perimeter, estimated time interval to arrival, and estimated return date of borrowed equipment, supplies, and/or personnel, etc.

5. EOC/County Warning Point: Each Healthcare Facility will participate in a weekly HFMAS radio test and an annual exercise that includes communicating to MedComm/ESF#8–Health and Medical a set of standardized data elements or indicators describing the Healthcare Facility's resource capacity. (See Exhibit A of this MOU for forms). MedComm/ESF#8–Health and Medical will serve as an information center for recording and disseminating the type and amount of available resources at each Healthcare Facility. During a disaster drill or actual disaster, each Healthcare Facility will report to MedComm/ESF#8–Health and Medical the current status of their indicators. (For a more detailed account of MedComm's/ESF#8–Health and Medical responsibilities, see "MedComm Requirements").

6. Healthcare Facility Indicators: Each Healthcare Facility shall track and collect a set of Healthcare Facility resource measures that are reported to the Hospital Command Post and MedComm/ESF8 during a Disaster drill or actual Disaster. The indicators are designed to catalogue Healthcare Facility resources that could be available for other Healthcare Facilities during a Disaster.

7. Documentation: During a Disaster, the Recipient Facility will accept and honor the Donor Facility's standard requisition forms. Documentation should detail the items involved in the transaction, condition of the material prior to the loan (if applicable), and the party responsible for the material.

8. Authorization: The Recipient Facility will have supervisory direction over the Donor Facility's staff, to the same extent that it supervises its own staff, once such staff report for duty to the Recipient Facility. Notwithstanding the foregoing, if the Donor Facility is the VA Hospital, it shall retain supervisory direction over its own staff.

9.   Communications: Healthcare Facilities will collaborate on the HMACS radio communication system to ensure a dedicated and reliable method to communicate with MedComm/ESF#8– Health and Medical and other Healthcare Facilities. A back-up conference call landline telephone system may be used as a semi-secure system for discussing sensitive information.

10.   Public Relations: Each Healthcare Facility is responsible for developing and coordinating with the other Healthcare Facilities and relevant organizations (EOC/JIC) the media response to a Disaster. This shall not preclude a Healthcare Facility from responding to media requests directed to such facility. Healthcare Facilities are encouraged to develop and coordinate the outline of their response prior to any disaster. Partner Facilities should be familiar with their partner's procedures for addressing the media.

11.   Emergency Management Committee Chairperson: Each Healthcare Facility's Emergency Management Committee Chairperson (i.e., Safety Committee, Environment of Care, etc.) is responsible for disseminating the information regarding this MOU to relevant Healthcare Facility personnel, coordinating and evaluating the Healthcare Facility's participation in exercises of the mutual aid system, and incorporating the material terms of this Memorandum into the Healthcare Facility's emergency management plan.

V.   General Principles Governing Medical Operations, the Transfer of Pharmaceuticals, Supplies or Equipment, or the Evacuation of Patients

1.   Partner Healthcare Facility: During a disaster, the Impacted Facility may first call its Partner Healthcare Facility for personnel or material assistance or to request the evacuation of patients to the Partner Healthcare Facility. The Donor Healthcare Facility will inform its Partner Facility of the degree and time frame in which it can meet the request.

2.   MedComm: The Recipient or Impacted Facility is responsible for notifying and informing MedComm of its personnel or material needs or its need to evacuate patients and the degree to which its Partner Healthcare Facility is unable to meet these needs. Prior to the activation of ESF#8–Health and Medical, the senior administrator or designee of the Impacted Facility will contact the other participating Healthcare Facilities via MedComm to determine the availability of additional personnel or material resources, including the availability of beds, as required by the situation. The Recipient Facility will be informed as to which Healthcare Facilities should be contacted directly for assistance that has been offered. The senior administrator/Incident Commander (or designee) of the Recipient or Patient-Transferring Facility will coordinate directly with the senior administrator (or designee) of the Donor or Patient-Accepting Facility for this assistance.

3.   Initiation of Transfer of Personnel, Material Resources, or Patients: Only the senior administrator/Incident Commander or designee at each Healthcare Facility has the authority to initiate the transfer or receipt of personnel, material resources, or patients.

      Personnel offered by Donor Facilities shall be fully accredited or credentialed by the Donor Facility. Donor Facilities may send resident physicians, medical/nursing and allied health students, or other persons in-training (referred to herein as "Staff In-Training") if agreed to by the Recipient Facility. Upon accepting Staff In-Training, the Recipient Facility agrees to provide adequate supervision for such Staff In-Training and to assign such Staff In-Training to duties consistent with their level of training and experience. Notwithstanding the foregoing, if the Donor Facility is the VA Hospital, it will assign one of its own employees to provide adequate supervision over all VA Hospital employees. The identification badges of all donated individuals shall identify the Healthcare Facility through which they are employed, their professional discipline (e.g., RN, MD), and whether such individuals are Staff In-Training.

In the event of the evacuation of patients, the medical director of the Patient-Transferring Facility will notify the local fire/EMS department of its situation and seek assistance, if necessary. Additional assistance may be requested from private ambulance companies, local aero medical services, and other municipal private transporting services.

VI.   Specific Principles of Understanding

A.   Medical Operations/Loaning Personnel

1.   Communication of Request: The request for the transfer of personnel initially can be made verbally. The request, however, must be followed up with written documentation. The written request shall occur prior to the arrival of personnel at the Recipient Facility. The Recipient Facility will specify to the Donor Facility the following:

   a.   The type and number of requested personnel.
   b.   An estimate of how quickly the request is needed.
   c.   The location where they are to report.
   d.   An estimate of how long the personnel will be needed.
   e.   Any specialized training needs (i.e. WMD, ALS) for the personnel needed.

2.   Documentation: The donated personnel will be required to wear their Donor Facility identification badge at all times while at the Recipient Facility's. The Recipient Facility will be responsible for the following:

   a.   Meeting the arriving donated personnel.
   b.   Comparing the donated personnel's identification against the list of personnel provided by the Donor Facility and assuring it is physically apparent on the individual when working.
   c.   Providing additional identification, e.g., "visiting personnel" badge, to the arriving donated personnel.
   d.   Provide appropriate facility and operations orientation.

The Recipient Facility will accept the professional credentialing determination of the Donor Facility for those services for which the personnel are credentialed at the Donor Facility.

3.   Supervision: The Recipient Facility's senior administrator or designee shall identify where and to whom the donated personnel are to report. The Recipient Facility shall provide supervision for donated personnel to the same extent that it supervises its own staff. Notwithstanding the foregoing, if the Donor Facility is the VA Hospital, it will provide its own supervision for its employees. The Recipient Facility's supervisor or designee will meet the donated personnel or the personnel and its designated supervisor if the Donor Facility is the VA, at the point of entry of the facility and brief the donated personnel of the situation and their assignments. If appropriate, the "emergency staffing" rules of the Recipient Facility will govern assigned shifts. The donated personnel's shift, however, should not be longer than the customary length practiced at the Donor Facility.

4.   <u>Staff Support:</u> The Recipient Facility shall provide the Donor Facility personnel asked to work for extended periods of time and for multiple shifts with food, housing, and/or transportation similar to that provided for the Recipient Facility's regular staff. The costs associated with these forms of support will be the sole obligation of the Recipient Facility.

5.   <u>Salary Costs:</u> The Recipient Facility will reimburse the Donor Facility for the salaries of the donated personnel at the rate paid to such personnel by the Donor Facility. Notwithstanding the foregoing, all personnel provided by the Donor Facility shall remain at all times employees of the Donor Facility and the Donor Facility shall be solely responsible for paying the salaries/wages of such donated personnel. Reimbursement of the cost of salaries for the donated personnel will be made within ninety (90) days following the Recipient Facility's receipt of an invoice from the Donor Facility. If non-hospital based staff (i.e., agency RN) is provided, the Receiving Facility will directly pay the staffing agency for use of its personnel which reimbursement shall equal such agency's contracted rate.

6.   <u>Professional Credentialing:</u> Each Healthcare Facility shall establish a mechanism for granting emergency clinical privileges' for physicians, nurses, and other licensed healthcare providers to provide services at the Recipient Facility.

7.   <u>Demobilization Procedures:</u> The Recipient Facility will provide and coordinate any necessary demobilization procedures and post-event stress debriefing. The Recipient Facility is responsible for providing the donated personnel transportation necessary for their return to the Donor Facility, if requested.

B.   Transfer of Pharmaceuticals, Supplies or Equipment

1.   <u>Communication of Request:</u> The request for the transfer of pharmaceuticals, supplies, or equipment initially can be made verbally. The request, however, shall be followed up with a written communication. The written request shall be sent to the Donor Facility prior to the receipt of any material resources at the Recipient Facility. The Recipient Facility will specify for the Donor Healthcare Facility the following:

    a.   The quantity and exact type of requested items.
    b.   An estimate of how quickly the request is needed.
    c.   Time period for which the supplies, equipment, and medications will be needed.
    d.   Location to which the supplies, equipment, and medications should be delivered.

    The Donor Facility will identify how long it will take it to fulfill the request and communicate same to Recipient Facility. Because response time is critical during a disaster response, each Healthcare Facility shall use its best efforts to respond to requests for supplies, pharmaceuticals or equipment quickly.

2.   <u>Documentation:</u> The Recipient Facility will honor the Donor Facility's standard order requisition form as documentation of the request and receipt of the materials. The Recipient Facility's designee will confirm the receipt of the resources provided. The documentation will detail the following:

    a.   The items provided.
    b.   The condition of the equipment prior to the loan (if applicable).
    c.   The responsible parties for the borrowed material.

The Donor Facility is responsible for tracking the borrowed inventory through its standard requisition forms. Upon the return of the equipment, etc., the original invoice will be co-signed by the senior administrator or designee of the Recipient Facility who shall record the condition of the borrowed equipment.

3.   Transporting of Pharmaceuticals, Supplies, or Equipment: The Recipient Facility is responsible for coordinating the transportation of materials both to and from the Donor Facility. This coordination may involve government and/or private organizations, and the Donor Facility may also offer transport. Upon request, the Recipient Facility must return the loaned items and pay the transportation fees for returning or replacing all such borrowed items.

4.   Care of Equipment and Supplies: The Recipient Facility is responsible for appropriate safeguarding, use, and maintenance of all borrowed pharmaceuticals, supplies, or equipment.

5.   Cost of Repair/Replacement: Each Healthcare Facility agrees that it shall reimburse a Donor Facility for any loss, damage or destruction of equipment which occurred while such equipment was in the possession or custody of such Healthcare Facility.

6.   Cost of Supplies. Each Healthcare Facility shall reimburse any Donor Facility for the cost of donated supplies and pharmaceuticals. Payment shall be made within ninety (90) days of Recipient Facility's receipt of an invoice from the Donor Facility.

7.   Demobilization Procedures: The Recipient Facility is responsible for the rehabilitation and prompt return of the borrowed equipment in working order to the Donor Facility.

C.   Transfer/Evacuation of Patients

1.   Communication of Request: The request for the transfer of patients initially can be made verbally. The request, however, must be followed up with a written communication prior to the actual transferring of any patients. The Patient-Transferring Facility will specify the following for the Patient-Accepting Facility:

a.   The number of patients needed to be transferred.
b.   The general condition of such patients.
c.   Any type of specialized services required (ICU bed, burn bed, trauma care, etc.).

2.   Documentation: The Patient-Transferring Facility is responsible for providing the Patient-Receiving Facility with the patient's complete medical records, insurance information and other patient information necessary for the care of the transferred patient. The Patient-Transferring Facility is responsible for tracking the destination of all patients transferred out.

3.   Transporting of Patients: The Patient-Transferring Facility is responsible for coordinating and financing the transportation of patients to the Patient-Receiving Facility. The Patient-Receiving Facility's senior administrator or designee will designate the point of entry. Once admitted, each patient becomes the Patient-Receiving Facility's patient and under the care of the Patient-Receiving Facility's admitting physician until discharged, transferred or reassigned. The Patient-Transferring Facility is responsible for transferring of extraordinary drugs or other special patient needs (e.g., equipment and blood products) along with the patient if requested by the Patient-Receiving Facility and subject to availability at the Patient-Transferring Facility. If the Donor Facility is the VA Hospital, its staff is excluded from providing transportation of patients pursuant to this paragraph.

4.   Admission: The Patient-Receiving Facility will designate the patient's admitting service, the admitting physician for each patient, and, if requested, will provide at least temporary courtesy privileges (including evaluation, treatment, and documentation) to the patient's original attending physician.

5.   Notification: The Patient-Transferring Facility is responsible for notifying the patient's family or guardian and the patient's attending or personal physician of the situation. The Patient-Receiving Facility may assist in notifying the patient's family and personal physician. Notification will be done in compliance with all state and federal privacy laws including, but not limited to, the Health Insurance Portability and Accountability Act of 1996 ("HIPPA") and in accordance with emergency declaration allowances.

D.   MedComm Function

The HMACS provides the means for the Healthcare Facilities to coordinate among themselves and as a unit to integrate with PBCEM, PBCHD, Police and EMS during a Disaster.

MedComm serves as the initial data center for collecting and disseminating current information about equipment, bed capacity and other Healthcare Facility resources during a Disaster. (See attached form) The information collected by the Communication Center is to be used only for Disaster preparedness and response. This responsibility will be shared or transferred to ESF#8–Health and Medical once it becomes operational.

In the event of a Disaster or during a Disaster drill, Healthcare Facilities will be prepared to provide the following information:

1.   Total number of injury victims its Emergency Department can accept, and if possible, the number of victims with minor and major injuries;

2.   Total number of operating beds available to accept patients in the following units:

a.	general medical (adult)	h.	pediatric intensive care
b.	general surgical (adult)	i.	burn
c.	general medical (pediatric)	j.	psychiatric
d.	general surgical (pediatric)	k.	sub acute care
e.	obstetrics	l.	skilled care beds
f.	cardiac intensive care	m.	operating suites
g.	neonatal intensive care		

3.   Total number of items available for loan or donation to another Healthcare Facility:

a.	respirators/ventilators (adult/pediatric)	i.	external pacemakers
		j.	designated medications
b.	IV infusion pumps	k.	bedside monitoring device
c.	dialysis machines	l.	monitor defibrillators
d.	hazmat decontaminat. equip.	m.	pulse ox
e.	Hazmat PPE	n.	transport equipment (stretcher, wheelchair, etc.)
f.	MRI		
g.	CT/PET scanner	o.	transport vehicles
h.	hyper baric chamber		

4.   The personnel in the following specialties currently available for loan to another Healthcare Facility (list to include special information such as training level of WMD, Certifications-ACLS, PALS, etc) and Vaccinations:

Physicians: **Registered Nurses:**
Anesthesiologists   Emergency
Emergency Medicine   Critical Care
General Surgeon   Operating Room
Infectious Disease   Pediatrics
OB-GYN   Med/Surg
Pediatricians   Occupational Health
Trauma Surgeons   Oncology/Hematology
Internal Medicine

Other Personnel:
Laboratory Personnel   Residents, Other Persons in Training
Maintenance Workers   Radiology Personnel
Mental Health Workers   Respiratory Therapists
Nurse Anesthetists   Plant Engineers
Nurse Practitioners   Security personnel
Physician Assistants   Social Workers
                                                     Others as indicated

VII.   Miscellaneous Provisions

A.   Term. The term of this MOU shall be for a period of three (3) years commencing on the _____ day of _____, and continuing in effect until the _____ day of _____. Thereafter, this MOU shall automatically renew for successive periods of one year unless sooner terminated as provided herein.

B.   Termination.

1.   This MOU may be terminated upon unanimous written agreement of the parties hereto.

Each party to this Memorandum may terminate its participation hereunder, with or without cause, by providing written notice to the other parties at least thirty (30) days prior to the effective date of such termination.

Notice. All notices required or allowed by this MOU shall be delivered by hand delivery or certified mail, return receipt requested, to the party to whom such notice is to be given at the following addresses:

All parties and address provided under Exhibit B

D.   Confidentiality. Each Healthcare Facility shall maintain the confidentiality of all patient health information and medical records in accordance with applicable state and federal laws, rules and regulations including, but not limited to, HIPAA.

E.   Insurance. Each Healthcare Facility shall maintain, at its sole cost and expense, professional liability insurance coverage for itself and its respective employees with: (a) a per claim limit of not less than the then current cap on damages in a medical malpractice suit, as set forth in Florida statutes and (b) an annual aggregate limit equal to two (2) times the amount of the required per claim limit set forth in item (a), above. Notwithstanding the foregoing, if the Donor Facility is the VA Hospital, insurance coverage is limited to that provided under the Federal Tort Claims Acts.

F.   <u>Liability</u>. No party shall assume any liability for any injury (including death) to any persons, any damage to any property or other claim arising out of the acts or omissions of any other party or parties or any of such other party's or parties' agents or employees.

G.   <u>Independent Contractors</u>. All parties, in the performance of their respective obligations under this Agreement, shall be acting in its own individual capacity and not as an agent, employee, partner, joint venturer or associate of the other parties. The employees and agents of one party shall not be deemed or construed to be the employees, agents or partners of the other parties for any purpose whatsoever. The parties expressly understand and agree that each party is an independent contractor of the other parties and that no party to this Agreement is authorized to bind the any other party to any liability or obligation or to represent that it has any such authority.

H.   <u>Counterparts</u>. This Agreement may be executed in two or more counterparts, all of which shall, in the aggregate, be considered one and the same instrument.

I.   <u>Cooperation Regarding Claims and Litigation</u>. The parties agree that to the extent permitted by their respective professional liability insurance programs, they shall provide each other with full cooperation in assisting each other, their duly authorized officers, employees, agents, representatives and attorneys, in investigating, defending or prosecuting incidents involving circumstances which occurred during the term of this Agreement and which relate to the duties and obligations described herein, including those which were not raised until after termination of this Agreement.

J.   <u>Release</u>. Each party agrees that it shall waive its right to pursue any claim or legal action against another party arising out of or relating to such other party's provision of staff, equipment, medications or supplies pursuant to this Memorandum, unless such other party has: (a) failed to use reasonable care in credentialing personnel provided under this Memorandum; (b) failed to use reasonable care in maintaining all equipment and supplies furnished hereunder; or (c) has acted with malice or engaged in an intentional wrongful act.

K.   By signing this Memorandum of Understanding each Healthcare Facility is evidencing its intent to abide by the terms of the MOU in the event of a medical disaster as described above. The terms of this MOU are to be incorporated into the Healthcare Facility's emergency management /disaster plans.

L.   Entire Agreement. This Agreement constitutes the entire understanding and agreement between the parties with regard to the subject matter hereof and supercedes all other negotiations, understandings and representations, if any, made by and between the parties.

IN WITNESS WHEREOF, the parties have executed this Agreement as of the date and year written below.

AG Holley
Boca Raton Community Hospital
Bethesda Memorial Hospital
Columbia Hospital
Delray Medical Center
Glades General Hospital
Good Samaritan Medical Center
JFK Medical Center
Jupiter Medical Center
Palm Beach Gardens
Palms West Hospital
St Mary's Medical Center
VA Medical Center
West Boca Medical Center
Wellington Regional Medical Center

EXHIBIT A

See Attached Forms:

PRIMARY DATA COLLECTION FORM

SECONDARY DATA COLLECTION FORMS

PRIMARY DATA COLLECTION FORM

In the event of an emergency, record the time of communication, the total number of injury victims the receiving Healthcare Facility can accept, and, if possible, the number of major* and minor* * injury victims the Healthcare Facility can accept.

Date:

Page #:

Hospital	Phone/Fax	Time	Total Number Patients	Minor Injuries	Major Injuries	Comments
Bethesda Memorial Hospital	ph: fax:					
Boca Raton Community Hospital	ph: fax:					
Columbia Hospital	ph: fax:					
Delray Medical Center	ph: fax:					
Glades General Hospital	ph: fax:					
Good Samaritan Medical Center	ph: fax:					
JFK Medical Center	ph: fax:					
Jupiter Medical Center	ph: fax:					
Palm Beach Gardens Medical Center	ph: fax:					
Palms West Hospital	ph: fax:					
St Mary's Medical Center	ph: fax:					
VA Medical Center	ph: fax:					
Wellington Regional Medical Center	ph: fax					
West Boca Medical Center	ph: fax					

* "Major injury victims": those expected to require admission and/or significant medical/ hospital resources (operating room, critical care, extensive orthopedics intervention, etc.)
** "Minor injury victims": those expected to be treated and released or require very little medical/ hospital resources.

SECONDARY DATA COLLECTION FORM *

If time or need permits, request the following information from the donating Healthcare Facility.

Healthcare Facility Name:
Facility Phone and Fax #:
Person Completing Form:
Person Authorizing Assistance:
Date and Time:

Number of Open/Available Beds/Time		Total Available to Donate/ Time	
General medical (adult)		Respirators/Ventilators (adult/pediatric)	
General surgical (adult)		IV Infusion Pumps	
General medical (pediatric)		Dialysis Machines	
General surgical (pediatric)		Hazmat Decon. Equipment	
Obstetrics		Hazmat PPE	
Cardiac ICU		MRI	
NICU		CT Scanner	
PICU		Hyper baric Chamber	
Burn		External Pacemakers	
Psychiatric		Designated Medications (specify)	
Trauma		Bedside Monitoring Devices	
OR Suites		Monitor/Defibrillators	
Skilled Nursing & Sub acute Care		Pulse OX/ETCO2	
		Transport Equipment (stretcher, wheelchairs)	

* During an actual disaster or disaster drill, hospitals should complete the above form with the most current information available and have this information ready for dissemination to the EOC, requesting hospitals, and the HMAC MedComm.

SECONDARY DATA COLLECTION FORM *

Healthcare Facility Name:
Facility Phone and Fax #:
Person Completing Form:
Person Authorizing Assistance:
Date and Time:

Physician	Number of Personnel Currently Available to Loan/Donate to Partner Hospital*/ Time	Specialized Certifications and Vaccination Coverage**
Anesthesiology		
Emergency Medicine		
General Surgeon		
General Medicine		
OB-GYN		
Pediatrician		
Trauma Surgeon		
Other as indicated		
Registered Nurses		
Emergency		
Critical Care		
Operating Room		
Pediatrics		
Other as indicated		
Other Personnel		
Laboratory Personnel		
Maintenance Workers		
Mental Health Workers		
Nurse Anesthetists		
Nurse Practitioners		
Physician Assistants		
Radiology Personnel		
Residents/Other Persons In Training		
Respiratory Therapists		
Plant Engineers		
Security Personnel		
Social Workers		
Others as indicated		

* During an actual disaster or disaster drill, hospitals should complete the above form with the most current information available and have this information ready for dissemination to local fire/EMS, requesting healthcare facilities, and the HMACS MedComm.
** SKILLS KEY: A-ACLS, C-CISD P-PALS, H1-HAZMAT AWARE, H2-HAZMAT TECHNICAL.

EXHIBIT B

Gary Strack, CEO
Boca Raton Community Hospital
800 Meadows Road
Boca Raton, FL 33486

Robert Hill, CEO
Bethesda Memorial Hospital
2815 South Seacrest Boulevard
Boynton Beach, FL 33435

Valerie Jackson, CEO
Columbia Hospital
2201 45th Street
West Palm Beach, FL 33407

Mitch Feldman, CEO
Delray Medical Center
5352 Linton Boulevard
Delray Beach, FL 33484

Dan Aranda, CEO
Glades General Hospital
1201 South Main Street
Belle Glade, FL 33430

Mary Bazzicaluto, COO
Good Samaritan Medical Center
1300 North Flagler Drive
West Palm Beach, FL 33402

Phil Robinson, CEO
JFK Medical Center
5301 South Congress Avenue
Atlantis, FL 33462

Michael Barry, CEO
Jupiter Medical Center
1210 South Old Dixie Highway
Jupiter, FL 33458

Mary Jo Gregory, CEO
Palm Beach Gardens Medical Center
3360 Burns Road
Palm Beach Gardens, FL 33410

Heather Rohan, CEO
Palms West Hospital
13001 Southern Boulevard
Loxahatchee, FL 33470

Peter Marmerstein, CEO
St. Mary's Medical Center
901 45th Street
West Palm Beach, FL 33407

Walt Mickens, CEO
West Boca Medical Center
21644 State Road 7
Boca Raton, FL 33428

Kevin DiLallo, CEO
Wellington Regional Medical Center
10101 Forest Hill Boulevard
West Palm Beach, FL 33414

Bill Farrell, Chairman
Healthcare Emergency Response Coalition
c/o Palm Beach County Medical Society
3540 Forest Hill Blvd, Suite 101
West Palm Beach, FL 33406

Appendix C

Operational Guidelines or Bylaws (Sample)

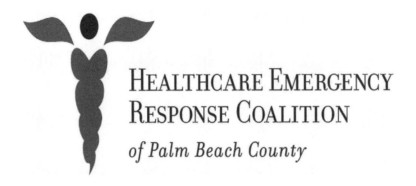

OPERATIONS GUIDELINES

LAST REVISED
2010

NAME

The name of the organization shall be the Healthcare Emergency Response Coalition of Palm Beach County hereafter referred to as HERC.

MISSION

To develop and promote the healthcare emergency preparedness and response capabilities of Palm Beach County.

PURPOSE

1. Provide a forum for the healthcare community to interact with one another and other response agencies at a county, regional, and state level to promote emergency preparedness.

2. Coordinate and improve the delivery of healthcare emergency response services.

3. Foster communication between local, regional, and state entities on community-wide emergency planning and response.

4. Ensuring overall readiness through coordination of community-wide training and exercises.

5. Promote preparedness in the healthcare community through standardized practices and integration with other response partners.

COMPOSITION OF COALITION

GENERAL MEMBERSHIP

Membership in the Coalition shall be extended to the following agencies, institutions, and community-wide emergency response related disciplines within Palm Beach County:

- Lead Agency for ESF 4—Fire Fighting—Palm Beach County Fire Rescue
- Lead Agency for ESF 6—Mass Care—American Red Cross
- Lead Agency for ESF 8—Health and Medical—Palm Beach County Health Department
- Lead Agency for ESF 16—Law Enforcement—Palm Beach County Sheriff
- Support Agency for ESF 8—Health Care District of Palm Beach County
- Support Agency for ESF 8—Palm Beach County Medical Society

- Palm Beach County Hospitals
- Palm Beach County Emergency Management
- Region 7 Chair

Voting members who represent individual disciplines and geographic interests on community-wide emergency planning and response matters, identify issues related to regional planning response matters, propose solutions to identified problem areas and seek to establish interdisciplinary consensus on response practices and procedures to be utilized by all HERC members.

DESIGNATED REPRESENTATIVE

The appointing authority of each HERC Member shall designate a representative to attend and vote at HERC meetings. The representative should have a role at the hospital/agency related to emergency preparedness or disaster response.

ALTERNATES REPRESENTATIVES

Each appointing authority shall designate two alternate representatives either of whom can attend and vote at a meeting at which the Designated Representative cannot be present. The representatives should have a role at the hospital/agency related to emergency preparedness or disaster response. For hospitals, it is recommended either the Designated Representative or one of the Alternate Representatives should be the hospital's Infection Control Practitioner.

TERM

The appointing authority shall determine the term of office for each representative.

VACANCIES

The appointing authority shall be advised of any vacancy and asked to appoint a replacement.

CONFIRMATION

All representatives and alternates must be reviewed by chairperson and presented for approval to the Steering Committee with a recommendation for vote.

TRUSTED PARTNERS

In addition, HERC shall recognize the Palm Healthcare Foundation as a founding partner and the following groups as TRUSTED PARTNERS:

- Private EMS Transport
- Metropolitan Medical Response System (MMRS)
- Medical Examiners
- Funeral Home Directors
- Mental Health Professionals
- Pharmacies
- Medical labs
- Military (National Guard)
- Salvation Army
- Amateur Radio Operators
- Veterinarians
- Florida Hospital Association
- South Florida Hospital and Healthcare Association
- Dental Profession
- Treasure Coast Health Council
- The School District of Palm Beach County
- School Nurse Program—Health Department and Health Care District
- Nursing Home Association

TRUSTED PARTNERS will be invited to attend meetings and receive copies of agendas and minutes. However, they will be non-voting members.

REGULAR MEETINGS

Regular meetings of the HERC shall be held monthly unless modified by the Chairperson. Each meeting shall follow a predetermined agenda established by the Chairman in consultation with the Steering Committee. Minutes of the meeting shall be taken and retained for a period of not less than five (5) years. The minutes will be posted on the HERC website 5 business days prior to the next meeting.

SPECIAL MEETINGS

Special meetings may be held upon call of the Chairperson or at the request of any two Steering Committee members. Minutes of the meeting shall be taken and retained for a period not less than five (5) years. The minutes will be posted on the HERC website 5 business days prior to the next meeting.

NOTICE

Written/Internet notice shall be provided of all regularly scheduled HERC Meetings at least five (5) working days prior to the meeting date. In the case of a Special Meeting, such notice shall state the purpose of the meeting. Special Meeting notices shall be not less than 24 hours.

QUORUM

A majority of General Membership representatives shall constitute a quorum for transaction of business.

VOTING

At any meeting having a quorum, action may be taken by a simple majority of those General Membership representatives who are present. If a quorum is not present at a meeting, transaction of business will take place under the condition that any motions that are put forth to a vote will be presented to absent voting representatives via electronic mail in order to receive a quorum vote. A reasonable amount of time will be allowed for receipt of absentee votes not to exceed ten days from the date of the meeting. If a quorum is not obtained the motion fails.

OPEN MEETINGS

Meetings shall not be open to the public or the press and media except when topics warranting their attendance will be discussed.

PARLIMENTARY PROCEDURE

Robert's Rules of Order will be used to guide the conduct of any meeting of the HERC.

STEERING COMMITTEE

The Steering Committee shall consist of the representatives of each of the following HERC Members and the Region 7 Health and Medical Co-Chairs:

- Chairperson—Representative from one of the Palm Beach County Hospitals
- Immediate Past Chairperson—Representative from one of the Palm Beach County Hospitals
- Vice Chairperson—Representative from the Lead Agency for ESF 8—Health Department
- Treasurer—Representative from one of the Palm Beach County Hospitals

- Secretary—Representative from one of the Palm Beach County Hospitals
- Education / Exercise Committee Chair—Representative from one of the Palm Beach County Hospitals
- Syndromic Surveillance Committee Chair—Representative from one of the Palm Beach County Hospitals who is an Infection Control Practitioner
- Communications Committee Chair—Representative from one of the Palm Beach County Hospitals
- HERC Representative from the Lead Agency for ESF 4—Palm Beach County Fire Rescue
- HERC Representative from the Lead Agency for ESF 16—Palm Beach County Sheriff
- HERC Representative from the Support Agency for ESF 8—Health Care District
- HERC Representative from the Support Agency for ESF 8—Medical Society
- HERC Representative from Palm Beach County Emergency Management
- The two Region 7 Health and Medical Co-Chairs

The Steering Committee shall determine issues the Coalition shall address, make recommendations to the Coalition membership on community-wide emergency related matters, coordinate the regional approach to community-wide emergency planning, training, and response, coordinate the fiscal matters for programs managed by the Coalition, and periodically ensure that the effectiveness of the Coalition is evaluated.

DUTIES OF STEERING COMMITTEE MEMBERS

CHAIRPERSON—The Chairperson shall provide the direction and leadership for the Coalition. He/she shall act as Chairperson of all Coalition meetings; serve as the official representative and spokesperson of the Coalition; act as the liaison to the Region 7 Domestic Security Terrorism Task Force Director and to other support foundations and agencies.

IMMEDIATE PAST CHAIRPERSON—The Immediate Past Chairperson shall provide transitional support to the Chairperson and Steering Committee, will be responsible for leading any strategic planning efforts, and participates as a full voting member of the Steering Committee.

VICE-CHAIRPERSON—The Vice-Chairperson shall preside over meetings in the absence of the Chairperson; serve as the liaison to outside agencies at the direction of the Chairperson; and perform other duties assigned by the Chairperson.

EDUCATION/EXERCISE COMMITTEE CHAIR—Tthe Education/Exercise Committee Chair shall preside over the Education/Exercise Committee which is tasked with researching and developing recommendations relating to purchasing of PPE and other associated equipment; recommending protocols to address regulatory issues; coordinating with regional and state activities relative to training and education; serving as a clearinghouse for training resources; and serving as the liaison with any tabletop exercises and live drills.

SYNDROMIC SURVEILLANCE COMMITTEE CHAIR—The Syndromic Surveillance Committee Chair shall be a hospital Infection Control Practitioner who will preside over the Syndromic Surveillance Committee which is tasked with coordinating with local, regional, and state efforts to implement a syndromic surveillance system in Palm Beach County.

COMMUNICATIONS COMMITTEE CHAIR—The Communications Committee Chair shall preside over the Communications Committee which is tasked with researching, planning, and coordinating all purchases of communications equipment (radio, telephone, internet, other) and MIR3 Notification System maintenance and activation as directed by the HERC Steering Committee and General Membership.

SECRETARY—The Secretary shall act as the liaison between HERC and the contracted administrative support staff approving written correspondence prior to distribution and assign and track the functions of the contracted administrative support staff. Tasks that the contracted administrative support staff will be responsible for include the production and distribution of agendas and minutes for HERC meetings including after action reports following drills and actual events, conduct surveys of HERC Membership as needed, coordinate training seminar registrations and RSVPs, maintain HERC records, provide support to HERC committees, maintain HERC Representative and Interested Party contact lists including email distribution list, and other administrative functions as needed.

TREASURER—The Treasurer shall work with the fiscal agent to coordinate the collection of membership dues along with any revenues associated with HERC activities, approve and track HERC financial matters in coordination with the Chair and fiscal agent, and will provide monthly reports to the Steering Committee and General Membership on the status of HERC account balances, revenues, and expenditures.

NON-TITLED STEERING COMMITTEE MEMBERS—The non-titled Steering Committee Members shall chair or sit on a standing committee, ad hoc committee, or task force.

REGULAR MEETINGS

Regular meetings of the Steering Committee shall be held monthly unless modified by the Chairperson. Each meeting shall follow a predetermined agenda established by the Chairman in consultation with the Steering Committee. Minutes of the meeting shall be taken and retained for a period of not less than five (5) years.

SPECIAL MEETINGS

Special meetings may be held upon call of the Chairperson or at the request of any two Steering Committee members. Minutes of the meeting shall be taken and retained for a period not less than five (5) years.

NOTICE

Written/Internet notice shall be provided of all regularly scheduled Steering Committee Meetings at least five (5) working days prior to the meeting date. In the case of a Special Meeting, such notice shall state the purpose of the meeting. Special Meeting notices shall be not less than 24 hours.

QUORUM

A majority of Steering Committee Members shall constitute a quorum for transaction of business.

VOTING

At any meeting having a quorum, action may be taken by a simple majority of those Steering Committee Members who are present. If a quorum is not present at a meeting, transaction of business will take place under the condition that any motions that are put forth to a vote will be presented to absent voting representatives via electronic mail in order to receive a quorum vote. A reasonable amount of time will be allowed for receipt of absentee votes not to exceed ten days from the date of the meeting. If a quorum is not obtained the motion fails.

OPEN MEETINGS

Meetings shall not be open to the public. Invited guests must be approved by the Chairperson or the Steering Committee prior to attendance.

PARLIMENTARY PROCEDURE

Robert's Rules of Order will be used to guide the conduct of any meeting of the HERC.

TENURE OF OFFICE

ELECTED POSITIONS—The tenure of office for the Chairperson and the Steering Committee's two elected hospital representatives shall commence in January of the calendar year following their election upon confirmation by the Steering Committee at the January Regular Steering Committee Meeting.

- CHAIRPERSON—shall serve for a term of one (1) year. The Chairperson may serve 2 consecutive one year terms.

- ELECTED HOSPTIAL REPRESENTATIVES—shall serve two year terms and will be limited to two consecutive terms.
- SECRETARY—shall serve for a term of (1) year.

APPOINTED POSITIONS—The tenure of office for the Immediate Past Chairperson, Vice-Chairperson, and all appointed non-titled Steering Committee Members shall commence in January following confirmation by the Steering Committee at the January Regular Steering Committee Meeting.

- IMMEDIATE PAST CHAIRPERSON—shall serve for a term of one (1) year for the year immediately following his or her term as Chairperson.
- VICE-CHAIRPERSON—shall serve for a term of one (1) year. The Vice-Chairperson will be the representative from the Lead Agency for ESF 8—Health Department
- APPOINTED NON-TITLED STEERING COMMITTEE MEMBERS—shall serve for a term of (1) year.

VACANCIES

Vacancies on the Steering Committee shall be appointed by the Chairperson and shall serve until the affected agency, institution, or discipline has selected their new representative.

EX-EFFICIO LIAISON REPRESENTATIVES

The Steering Committee may from time-to-time, elect to invite non-voting ex-officio representatives to associate with the HERC.

COMMITTEE STRUCTURE

STANDING COMMITTEES

The Standing Committees of HERC shall be the Communications Committee, the Education and Training Committee, and the Public Affairs and Finance Committee.

Syndromic Surveillance Committee—This Committee shall be chaired by a member of the Steering Committee who is a hospital Infection Control Practitioner who shall coordinate with local, regional, and state efforts to implement a syndromic surveillance system in Palm Beach County.

Communications Committee—This Committee shall be chaired by a member of the Steering Committee who shall research, plan, and coordinate all purchases of communications equipment (radio, telephone, internet, other) and MIR3 Notification System maintenance and activation as directed by the HERC Steering Committee and General Membership.

Education/Exercises Committee—This Committee shall be chaired by a member of the Steering Committee and shall research and develop recommendations relating to purchasing of PPE and other associated equipment; recommend protocols to address regulatory issues; coordinate with regional and state activities relative to training and education; serve as a clearinghouse for training resources; and serve as the liaison with any tabletop exercises and drills.

Public Affairs Committee—This Committee shall be chaired by a member of the Steering Committee and shall research and develop recommendations regarding legislative efforts and public relations.

AD HOC COMMITTEES

Ad Hoc Committees of HERC will be appointed by the Steering Committee as the need arises. Each Ad Hoc Committee will elect a chair and the life of the committee will be determined by the matter under consideration. The committee will be disbanded when the purpose has been served. The number of members will be determined by the Steering Committee.

TASK FORCES

Task Forces of HERC may be appointed by either the general membership or the Steering Committee as specific research/exploratory issues arise. Task Force member(s) will serve on a voluntary basis with the Chair appointed at time of establishment and will be disbanded when the purpose has been served.

ELECTIONS

Elections shall be held annually in December at the Regular General Membership HERC Meeting.

NOMINATIONS

ELECTED STEERING COMMITTEE MEMBERS—All elected Steering Committee Members must be nominated through the Coalition's nominating process as outlined in the Bylaws and determined by the Nominating Committee. Elected Members must be reviewed and confirmed by the Steering Committee at the January Regular Steering Committee Meeting.

APPOINTED STEERING COMMITTEE MEMBERS—All appointed Steering Committee Members shall be nominated by the appropriate appointing authority by virtue of their appointment to the Coalition and must be reviewed and confirmed by the Steering Committee at the January Regular Steering Committee Meeting.

NOMINATING COMMITTEE

A Nominating Ad Hoc Committee shall be created at the Regular September General Membership HERC Meeting. The Committee will be responsible for:

- Soliciting nominations for open elected positions from the Coalition
- Verifying eligibility and willingness to serve from each nominee
- Creating a list of nominees with names and biographical information and present said list to the General Membership at least fifteen (15) days prior to the date of the election
- Creating a ballot for the election at the December Regular General Membership HERC Meeting
- Tabulating votes and reporting the outcomes to the Coalition
- Members of the Nominating Committee shall be ineligible from serving on the Tellers Committee should they be on the ballot for any elected positions
- The ballot shall be approved by the Steering Committee prior to presentation to the General Membership

VOTING

Voting privileges shall be limited to General Membership Representatives or their Alternates. Voting shall be by written ballot. Simple majority shall elect. Only ballots received by the specified deadline shall be tabulated. In case of a tie, a run-off election by written ballot shall be held. In case of a second tie, the choice shall be by lot. Ballots shall be kept for thirteen (13) months after the election.

DISASTER PROVISIONS

In the event of a national disaster or other emergency situation that prevents HERC from fulfilling nominating, election, confirmation or other date sensitive activities, the Chairperson shall make arrangements for fulfilling the affected activity at a special meeting or via conference call, US postal mail, or electronic mail.

FISCAL AGENT

The Palm Beach County Medical Society Services shall be responsible for tracking all Coalition related expenditures directed by the General Membership. The record keeping shall be in accordance with Medical Society guidelines and generally accepted accounting practices.

Appendix D

Strategic Plan Using SWOT Methodology (Sample)

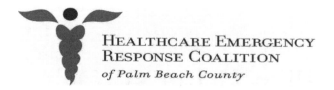

2007 Strategic Plan

Final (Year-End) Action Plan Update: 1/1/2008

Healthcare Emergency Response Coalition
of Palm Beach County, Florida

MISSION

To develop and promote the healthcare emergency preparedness, response, and recovery capabilities of Palm Beach County.

PURPOSE

- Provide a forum for the healthcare community to interact with one another and other response agencies at a county, regional, and state level to promote emergency preparedness.

- Coordinate and improve the delivery of healthcare emergency response services in collaboration with other stakeholders.

- Foster communication between local, regional, and state entities on community-wide emergency planning, response and recovery.

- Ensuring overall readiness through coordination of community-wide training and exercises.

- Promote preparedness in the healthcare community through standardized practices and integration with other response partners.

Sources of Pride for HERC members
(As identified in HERC strategic planning meeting of 11/17/2006)

1. Regular participation by member hospitals and agencies
2. Effective collaboration, participation and cooperation among all HERC members
3. Increased awareness of hospital planning and response needs by other HERC partners
4. Participation in outside regional and state meetings
5. Sharing the lessons learned by HERC with other Florida communities, as well as nationally and internationally
6. Continued funding support from Palm Health Foundation

Limitations which may prevent HERC from being more productive
(As identified in planning meeting of 11/17/2006)

1. Unequal work load distribution among a few members—same people are the only ones to volunteer
2. Partial loss of focus by the group on its real mission
3. Meetings not always focused or productive
4. Turnover among agency/hospital representatives
5. Lack of an orientation program for new members on their roles, responsibilities, and HERC operations
6. Lack of an orientation program for newly elected officers prior to taking office
7. Need for more clarity in roles, responsibilities, and authority of the following in the organizational operational guidelines:
   a. Steering Committee
   b. Standing committees
   c. Palm Beach Medical Society
   d. Disaster Coordinator
8. Need for bylaws to be revised to reflect new membership and provide additional operational guidance
9. Inconsistent performance in committees meeting and conducting their responsibilities
10. Lack of participation by Medical Examiner's Office in meetings

Tasks need to be completed
(As identified in planning meeting of 11/17/2006)

1. HERC team building
2. Expand HERC interested party membership:
   a. School District
   b. Behavioral Health Centers
3. Develop HERC membership manual
4. Complete Syndromic surveillance/ESSENCE implementation
5. Review/update HERC procedure including regional integration
6. Work on plans and procedures for
   a. Re-credentialing and licensing
   b. Medical surge capacity (including mass migration planning)
   c. Continuity of medical care (prehospital to hospital to outpatient support
   d. Recovery and COOP planning
   e. Communication
   f. Patient tracking plan
   g. Family Assistance Center
   h. Family Support Center
   i. Mass fatality planning with CME
   j. Internal hospital/agency plan
   k. External regional plan
   l. Increase media and public relations (including web page) efforts
   m. Behavioral health planning
   n. Utility loss planning
7. PPE updating and expand available inventory
8. Continue mass prophylaxis, SNS and CRI planning
9. Continue MRC planning and training
10. Courting support from elective officials

11. Continue work force support planning
12. Update HRSA needs assessment
13. Solicit additional support

Steps to Meet Strategic Goals
(As identified in planning meeting of 11/17/2006)

1. Complete a thorough review of the Operational Guidelines—1/28/07
2. Expand Interested Parties to include
    a. ESF 15 Volunteer Management
    b. ESF 19- Business and Industry
    c. Medical Reserve Corps
    d. Oakwood Mental Health and South County Mental Health
    e. Expand General membership to include School Board representative
3. Identifying HERC representative to serve on Palm Beach County Medical Society's Medical Services Board
4. Outline expectation for attendance at meeting by agency representatives and participation in committee activities
5. Secure a consistent meeting place that meets the needs of the organization - 12/15/06
    a. Large size
    b. Classroom style arrangement to promote communication
    c. Central location
6. Develop and publish a meeting schedule for 2007 calling for monthly 2-hour meetings of the General Membership and Steering Committee
7. Appoint committee chairs—12/15/06
    a. Consider splitting off Exercises to be separate committee or Ad Hoc committee
    b. Appoint personnel to standing committees—12/15/06
8. Develop an orientation manual for new members and elected officers—1/07
9. Complete final review of tasks to complete and develop action plan—1/07
10. Revise needed SOPs/policies and procedures—2/1/07
    a. Separate meeting—1/5/2007
    b. Ad hoc groups appointed to review and make needed changes to each procedure/policy/plan
    c. Changes approved by Steering Committee
11. Complete distribution of syndromic surveillance laptops to 40 designated recipients—12/15/06
12. Conduct well run General Membership meetings—ongoing
    a. Agenda created by Steering Committee and distributed before General Membership meeting
    b. Begin each General Membership meeting with Steering Committee report out
    c. Insure meetings focus is on decision making discussions and not simply information sharing
    d. information provided in the form of print summaries passed out before or during meeting
    e. Share the minutes from Steering Meetings with General Membership
    f. Increase use of Ad Hoc Committees and Task Forces

STRENGTHS, WEAKNESSES, THREATS, AND OPPORTUNITIES

Strengths	Weaknesses
Funding source: Palm Healthcare Foundation, regional grants	Turnover of membership
Different specialty perspectives	Meeting location at EOC
Realistic fear of unknown	Need for more focused and productive meetings
Using the work that has been completed to date	Need for clearer understanding of HERC roles and responsibilities
Embracing all response participants	Insufficient funding for equipment needs
Multi-disciplinary composition: public health, fire rescue, public safety	Better use of participants' time
Hospital perspective and needs being addressed	Too many varying commitments
Hurricane response support for one another	Missing potential partners (mental health and school board)
Driven membership and desire to succeed	Lack of hospital CEO interest and commitment
Technical support	Need to get the word out about our plans and resources
Different specialty perspectives	Lack of participation by Medical Examiner's Office
Using the work that has been completed to date	Overwhelming information demands
Presence of Dr. Lee and administrative support	

Opportunities	Threats
Secure more funding	Lack of focus; chasing too many opportunities
Be a model program	Divisive politics within HERC; attitude of some representatives who think in terms of "me, not we" or are critical instead of contributory
Improve profile with public	Complacency and stagnation
Do something concrete and demonstrable	Better mousetrap; someone else gets to JCAHO first; external competition
Increase inclusion by others like emergency management, CEMP, CERT, etc.	Perceived or actual failure during a real event
Get more exposure and interaction with elected officials and the state	Loss or reduction of internal support from HERC's organizational CEOs
Affiliate with a university, bringing national expertise to the table	
Expand cross-training with law enforcement (internal and external)	
Increase best practices model contributions to others in Florida, US, and international community	
Use our power in the political arena and increase our sphere of influence	
Attain real event success	
Have HERC representative on Palm Beach Medical Services Board	

HERC GOALS FOR 2007

Review "2007 Action Plan" (below) for HERC accomplishments in achieving the following eight primary goals for 2007.

1. **Stay true to the mission and purpose of HERC.**

2. **Make needed revisions to the Operational Guidelines.**

3. **Make needed revisions to current emergency planning and response procedures.**

4. **Ensure timely and effective communication between HERC members, Palm Beach County Medical Services Board, member CEOs and chief officers, elected officials, and the public.**

5. **Develop new response procedures including but not limited to:**

   a. **Communication**
   b. **Medical surge**
   c. **Fatality management**
   d. **Patient tracking**
   e. **Syndromic surveillance**
   f. **Behavioral and mental health Recovery**

6. **Continue to share the lessons learned in the operation of HERC with other interested communities through:**

   a. **Consulting**
   b. **Publishing articles**
   c. **Speaking at conferences**

7. **Initiate needed steps to ensure the sustainability of the organization (identify funding sources and ensure that needed funding support is obtained).**

8. **Complete implementation of Syndromic Surveillance program ESSENCE.**

2007 HERC ACTION PLAN

Goals	Description	HERC Action	Date Due	Responsible	Status
GOAL 1: Stay true to the mission and purpose of HERC		1. Appoint personnel to standing committees	1/1/07	Robbin Lee	Completed 100%
		2. Develop an orientation manual for new members	2/1/07	Claire Arnold	Pending
		3. Develop an orientation manual for new elected officers and committee members.	2/1/07	Claire Arnold	Pending
		4. Completing the tasks identified in the self assessment process of 11/2006 in accordance with this action plan developed by the Steering Committee and approved by the General Membership	6/1/2/07	Steering Committee	Completed 80%

Goals	Description	HERC Action	Date Due	Responsible	Status
GOAL 2: Make needed revisions to the organizational Operating Guidelines	Complete a thorough review of the Operational Guidelines	1. Expand Interested Parties to include:			
		• ESF 15 Volunteer Management (United Way)	5/18/07	Tenna Wiles	In process
		• ESF18– Business and Industry	5/18/07	Tenna Wiles	In process
		• Medical Reserve Corps	5/18/07	Jay Lee	In process
		• Oakwood Mental Health	5/18/07	Jay Lee	Completed
		• South County Mental Health	5/18/07	Jay Lee	In process
		• Non-governmental health clinics	5/18/07	Jay Lee	In process
		• School Board representative	5/18/07	Jay Lee	In process
				Sally Waite	Pending
		• Universities			
		Nova	5/18/07	Jay Lee	Completed
		FAU	5/18/07	Mark Goldstein	Completed
		USF	5/18/07	Michael Self	Pending
		2. Identify HERC representative to serve on Palm Beach County Medical Society's Medical Services Board	2/1/07	Tenna Wiles	Completed 100% (Russell, Lee on Board)
		3. Outline expectations for attendance at meetings by agency representatives and participating in committee activities			Pending: see goal 1, #3

Goals	Description	HERC Action	Date Due	Responsible	Status
GOAL 3: Make needed revisions in the current hospital planning and response procedures	Work on plans for: • Recredentialing and licensing • Medical surge capacity (incl. mass migration planning) • Continuity of medical care • Recovery and COOP planning: Communication Patient tracking plan Family Assistance Center Family Support Center Mass fatality planning with CME Internal hospital/agency plan External regional plan Increase media and public relations (e.g., web page) efforts Behavioral health planning Utility loss planning	1. Revise needed SOPs/policies and procedures 2. Separate meeting— January 5 2007 3. Appropriate committee/s appointed to review and make needed changes to each procedure and policy 4. Changes approved by Steering Committee and General Membership	5/18/07 1/5/07 2/1/07 On-going	Brenda Atkins and Workgroup Mary Russell Brenda Atkins Robbin Lee/ Steering Committee	Completed 100% Completed Completed Completed in part; in process

Goals	Description	HERC Action	Date Due	Responsible	Status
GOAL 4: Ensure timely and effective communication between HERC members, Palm Beach County Medical Services Board, member CEOs/chief officers, elected officials, and the public	Execute effective ongoing internal communication plan and external public relations plan	1. Secure a consistent meeting place that meets the needs of the organization: large size, classroom-style arrangement to promote communication, central location	12/15/06	Steering Committee	Completed 12/15/07
		2. Develop and publish a meeting schedule for 2007 calling for monthly 2-hour meetings of the General Membership and Steering Committee		Steering Committee	Completed 1/1/2007
		3. Appoint committee chairs—12/15/06 (split off exercises to be separate committee or ad hoc committee)		Steering Committee	Completed 2/2007
		4. Conduct well-run General Membership meetings: • Distribute agenda prior to meeting • Begin each meeting with Steering Committee report • Focus on decision making and not simply information sharing • Provide information in the form of printed summaries before or during meeting • Share Steering Meetings minutes • Increase use of ad hoc committees and task forces		Steering Committee	Completed and ongoing
		5. Complete and execute Public Relations Plan			Completed

Goals	Description	HERC Action	Date Due	Responsible	Status
GOAL 5: Develop new emergency response procedures		Actions include but are not limited to: 1. Communication 2. Medical surge 3. Fatality management 4. Patient tracking 5. Syndromic surveillance 6. Behavioral and mental health	9/1/07	Brenda Atkins	Pending
GOAL 6: Continue to share the lessons learned in the operation of HERC with other interested communities	Provide educational presentations and written information on HERC to both membership agencies and other external interested parties	Include outreach to: 1. Legislative and political leaders 2. FL Medical Association 3. FL Hospital Associations 4. State Government Officials HRSA, Emergency Management 5. Federal Agencies (HHS) 6. PBC Hospital CEOs	Done Done Done Done Done Pending	Tenna Wiles and Public Relations Committee	Completed Completed Completed Completed Completed Completed
GOAL 7: Initiate needed steps to ensure the sustainability of the organization	Ensure needed funding support for long-term sustainability for HERC	1. Identify current funding opportunities 2. Submit 3 grants in 2007 3. Acquire 1 NEW funding source for 2008	7/1/2007 10/1/2007 12/1/2007	John Brandt and Sustainability Workgroup	On-going Completed Completed (HHS grant Region VII PortBlue)

Goals	Description	HERC Action	Date Due	Responsible	Status
GOAL 8: Complete implementation of Syndromic Surveillance program ESSENCE by 14 hospital members	Syndromic Surveillance Committee Responsible to execute	1. Complete distribution of syndromic surveillance laptops to 40 designated recipients	12/15/06	Cindy Lang and Syndromic Surveillance Committee	Completed 1/1/2007
		2. Secure MOU from 14 of 15 membership	8/1/07		Pending 4 of 14 hospitals current using ESSENCE system
		3. Provide related training			
		4. Monitor and report performance			

About the Authors

Jay Lee (1948–2010) was the director for disaster services at the Palm Beach County Medical Society in West Palm Beach, providing administrative support to the Healthcare Emergency Response Coalition. In addition, he coordinated the Medical Reserve Corps and the special medical response team (SMRT) for Palm Beach County. In his thirty years of experience, he consulted with more than a hundred diverse organizations in a variety of areas, including behavioral healthcare, critical incident stress debriefing, psychological trauma management, human resources, disaster planning and response, and employee assistance programs. He published more than twenty articles and books on a wide variety of healthcare issues. He also served as an instructor for the FBI Medical Services, as an adjunct faculty member at Lynn University and NOVA University, and as the chief operating officer of Osprey Health Care, the largest behavioral health independent provider network in Florida.

Thomas W. Cleare serves as the administrator of health services and outreach for the Health Care District of Palm Beach County and is a former member of the steering committee of the Healthcare Emergency Response Coalition (HERC) in Palm Beach County. He has authored a number of articles dedicated to emergency preparedness and HERC and has presented at several national conferences on health policy topics, including emergency preparedness and community coalition sustainability. He previously served as administrative and planning support for Palm Beach County's HERC and was actively involved in its development and sustainability.

Mary Russell works under contract with the Florida Department of Health's Office of Public Health Preparedness as a senior hospital project manager for hospital preparedness projects. She has served as an emergency preparedness coordinator for Boca Raton Community Hospital, as chair of the Healthcare Emergency Response Coalition (HERC) of Palm Beach County, and as a steering committee and general committee member of HERC since 2003. She is also an active volunteer for the Palm Beach County Chapter of the Medical Reserve Corps.